HOME DETOX

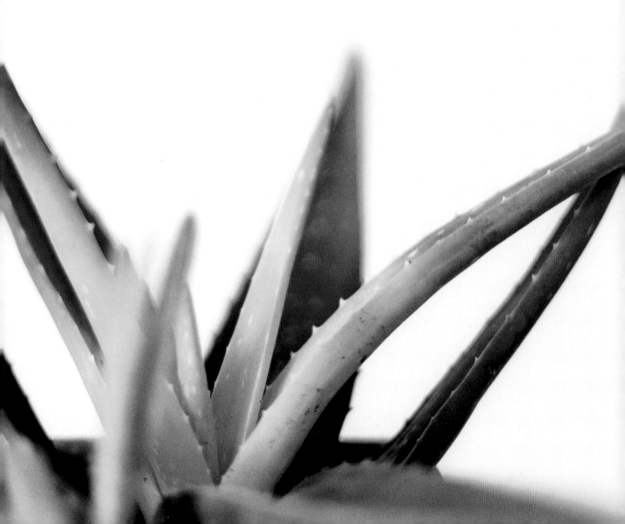

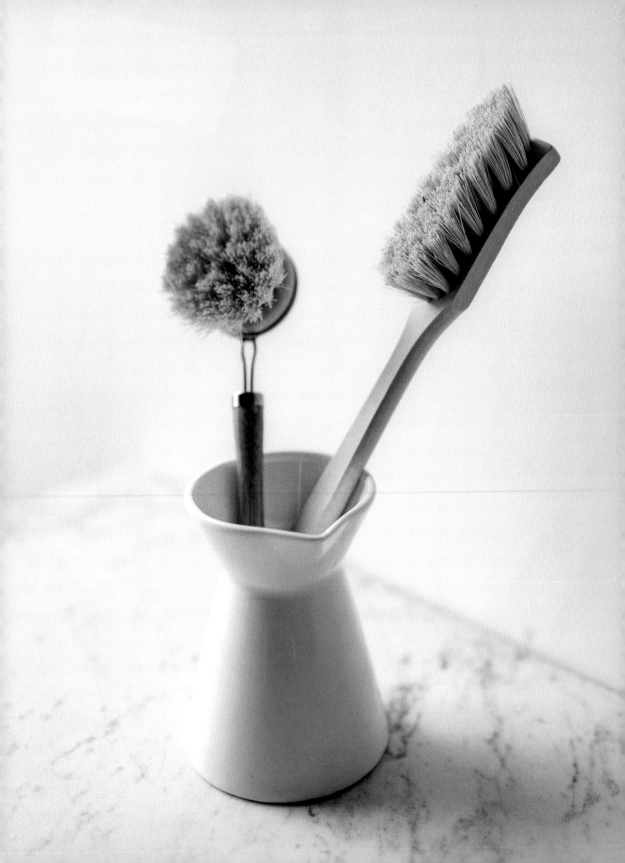

HOME
DETOX

MAKE YOUR HOME A HEALTHIER PLACE
FOR EVERYONE WHO LIVES THERE

Identify and eliminate hidden toxins

Combat common health problems

Clean away toxins in every room

Make your own cleaning solutions

DANIELLA CHACE, MSc, CN
FOREWORD BY JOEL FUHRMAN, MD

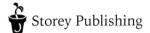
Storey Publishing

The mission of Storey Publishing is to serve our customers by publishing practical information that encourages personal independence in harmony with the environment.

Edited by Liz Bevilacqua
Art direction and book design by Michaela Jebb
Text production by Liseann Karandisecky
Indexed by Samantha Miller

Cover photography courtesy of Helen Milan Home
Interior photography by © John Gruen, 24, 27, 37, 49, 61, 65, 68, 71, 72, 75, 88, 95 (t.), 98, 102, 105, 111, 137 and Mars Vilaubi
    © Storey Publishing, LLC, ii, vi, ix, 8, 12, 29, 30, 41, 45, 51, 56, 76, 80, 83, 87, 89, 106, 127, 128, 134
Additional photography credits on page 195

Illustrations by © Daniella Chace, except © Artishokcs/Dreamstime.com, v & throughout (dots); © Blankstock/iStock.com,
    back cover (mattress); Michaela Jebb © Storey Publishing, LLC, back cover (nonstick pan); © Peacefully7/iStock.com,
    back cover (air freshener); © Vector/iStock.com, back cover (shower curtain)

Logos by © Environmental Working Group, www.ewg.org, 6; Fair Trade Certified, 74; GreenGuard Gold, 74; Lori Wyman,
    GOTS Representative in North America, 74; © MADE SAFE, a program of Nontoxic Certified 501(c)3, 74; STANDARD 100 by
    OEKO-TEX®, 74. Please note these organizations are not endorsing the text in this book and all logos are used for illustrative
    purposes only.

Text © 2023 by Daniella Chace

Storey books are available at special discounts when purchased in bulk for premiums and sales promotions as well as for fund-raising or educational use. Special editions or book excerpts can also be created to specification. For details, please call 800-827-8673, or send an email to sales@storey.com.

Storey Publishing
210 MASS MoCA Way
North Adams, MA 01247
storey.com

Printed in China through World Print
10 9 8 7 6 5 4 3 2 1

Library of Congress Cataloging-in-Publication Data on file

Dedicated to

RILEY REVALLIER, my stalwart research assistant, who is truly living an eco-lifestyle for health and planet

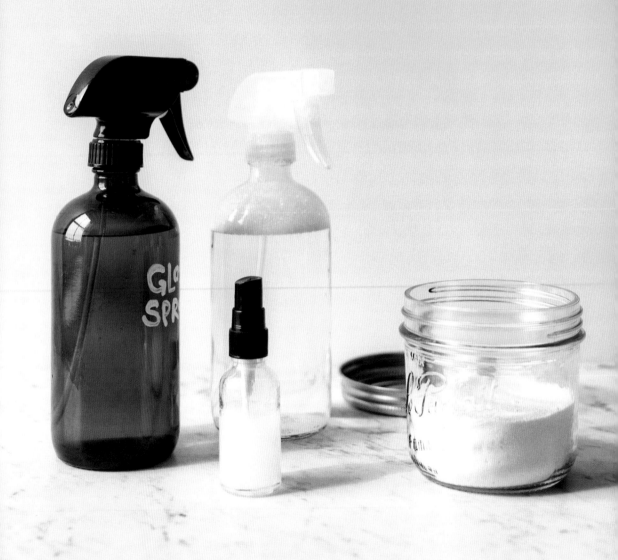

CONTENTS

Foreword by Joel Fuhrman, MD **VIII**

FOREWORD

In our modern lives, there are many sources of chemicals and toxic elements that can interfere with maintaining excellent health. We need to be aware of this now more than ever. Good nutrition, adequate sleep, and regular exercise are sometimes still not enough to resolve symptoms and restore health. The detective work to uncover causes of poor health must include environmental toxins and sensitivities to these toxins. Many people have realized the importance of minimizing dietary exposure to chemical toxins. However, it is also an unforgiving reality that our homes can be a source of toxic compounds that can contribute to symptomatic health conditions.

Daniella Chace has not only thoroughly researched these issues but also supplied the practical advice we need to keep our homes safe. Now, with this book, we have a guide for taking control of our health that addresses the hidden toxins in our homes.

It's important to realize that our exposure to toxins increases our risk for health problems. The likelihood that we, as individuals, will become ill from exposure depends largely on the types of toxins, the variety, and the length of exposure. In recent years we have become more knowledgeable about the fact that our homes contain elements that complicate our biological processes in ways that interfere with healing and can perpetuate illness.

One common, and ultimately most significant, way that these exposures affect our health is in their ability to cause inflammation. Inflammation can happen when foreign substances enter the bloodstream, and the immune system reacts by rushing aid to the location of the invader. However, chronic exposure can lead to chronic inflammation, which can worsen and perpetuate chronic disease such as autoimmune diseases and even increase risk of cancer. By eliminating chronic exposures, many cases of these types of disease could be avoided and the healing power of our bodies enhanced. It is also worth mentioning that some common hazardous household contaminants can damage DNA in ways that lead to premature aging and overall reduced life span.

Although the research is clear in making the connection between toxicity and human health risks, the answers have not always been straightforward. Daniella Chace provides answers to our modern questions. This book offers a well-researched program and a practical guide to help us locate the sources of toxins that carry the highest risk in our homes today. This is a daunting job, as the average home contains many thousands of items, each needing to be vetted for their various ingredients and materials. Taking the steps to remediate toxicity reduces the burden on our bodies and allows biological processes to function properly. Those who don't have an awareness of these negative health impacts and the sources of toxins in our homes won't stand a chance in avoiding them.

This book has the potential to help millions of people prevent exposure and subsequently illness. Simply put, removing the things that cause illness is a way to allow self-healing, to avoid needless suffering, and to improve quality of life. The goal of cleaner living is a worthwhile effort. This book offers an important contribution to improve your health, and to take a positive step toward the health of the planet to protect future generations.

— Joel Fuhrman, MD
#1 New York Times best-selling author of *Eat to Live*

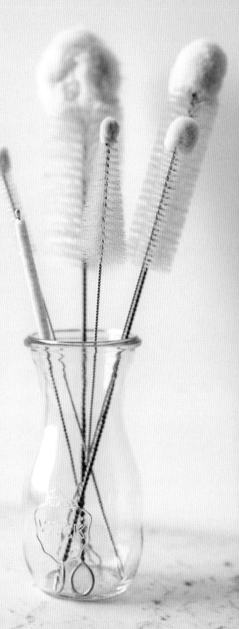

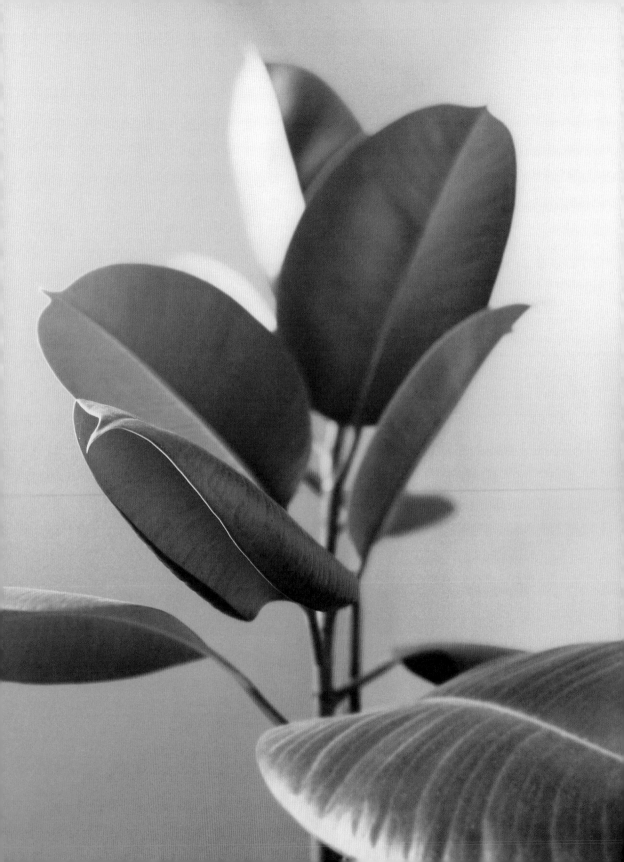

INTRODUCTION

OUR HOMES AND OUR HEALTH

In my work tracking down the triggers of disease, I have discovered that most are right under our noses. In fact, we are exposed to more toxins indoors than out. Our homes have become our number one source of toxicity, according to the US Environmental Protection Agency (EPA). Our indoor air can be two to five times more polluted than the air outside. One reason for this is that more than 40,000 chemicals are used to manufacture common consumer goods. Because we spend most of our time indoors, we are exposed to these chemicals daily, and they have a greater impact on our health than outdoor environmental pollution.

A PATH TO HEALTH

WELCOME TO A WHOLE NEW WORLD of insight into the causes of disease and a direct path to improved health. In my career as a toxicology clinician, I have been fortunate to help thousands of clients stem the devastating effects of environmental toxins. I draw from that experience to take you through a simple program to remove toxins from your home.

As a health practitioner, I work closely with my clients to make incremental changes with the goal of improving health issues and helping them feel strong and energetic. I have learned that the most direct route to this healthy state is through eating a diet rich in plant foods and removing toxins from the home that cause disease. My home detox program offers the actionable steps that have had the greatest positive impact for my clients through the years.

Many people reach out to me after their doctor has told them that they have a degenerative or chronic disease and there is nothing much to be done about it. The truth is that our bodies are making new cells around the clock, so we are constantly healing. When someone comes to me with a chronic illness, I use lab tests to evaluate urine, stool, and blood to look for nutrient deficiencies, infections, and toxins in the body. I often discover elevated levels of heavy metals, pesticides, phthalates, immune-suppressing fungi, or pathogenic bacteria. Then we get to work boosting nutrients, treating infections, and removing toxins. With

each small change, we are correcting imbalances and restoring health.

Toxins are linked to thousands of common health conditions and diseases. Polytetrafluoroethylene (PTFE)-treated substances from nonstick coatings on cooking pans (like Teflon) can raise cholesterol levels. Heavy metals can affect blood pressure. Volatile organic compounds (VOCs) can cause migraines. Rest assured, our bodies have a powerful natural detoxification system, enlisting the liver, kidneys, lungs, lymph, gastrointestinal tract, and even our sweat to excrete toxins. Our bodies are always actively working to remove harmful substances. We are miraculous this way. As soon as the compounds that are interfering with our biological processes are cleaned out, our bodies can begin to heal.

Whether members of your household are currently experiencing illness, or you are thinking ahead about protection from disease, removing toxins from your home supports prevention and lasting health. The first step in removing toxins is locating them, which is the heart of the program. Each recommendation is a step we would take together if I were right there with you in your home. This is a method for removing toxins and a path toward a nontoxic lifestyle. My wish is that you will feel the joy and power that comes with taking control and making changes that improve your well-being. I hope that you will soon be feeling the benefits of living a nontoxic life.

TOXINS ARE EVERYWHERE

WE ARE EXPOSED to toxins through items we touch, like clothes and toys, and through products we put on our skin, like lotions and perfume. We sit in disruptive electrical fields emitted from our modems, cell phones, and other devices. We breathe in noxious gases and airborne spores. We ingest toxins with our food, such as plastic from cutting boards. And one of the most surprising and common ways we take in toxins is by breathing in chemicals that have become stuck to the dust that permeates our indoor environments.

This consistent exposure to a combination of toxic substances can overwhelm our immune systems and interfere with biological functions. For example, studies have proven that chronic low exposures to common VOCs may be a significant health issue. VOCs are found in items that we come in contact with daily, such as oil-based paints, paint strippers, nail polish remover, adhesives, wood finishes, Teflon-coated pans, and air fresheners. They arise from specific chemicals used in those products, including acetaldehyde, acetone, formaldehyde, hexane, and toluene, and evaporate into the air in our homes. They wreak havoc on the inner workings of our cells; they can stop cells from replicating properly, interfere with cellular repair and development, and reduce the ability to make energy efficiently. Daily exposure to common household items that emit VOCs can promote the development of health conditions such as chronic fatigue syndrome, premature aging, and cancer.

BECOME A TOXIN DETECTIVE

I WILL SHOW YOU HOW to find hidden sources of toxins, remove them, and avoid bringing others into your home. My clients often notice quick improvement in their symptoms after they've removed a trigger from their home. As you learn more about how toxins interfere with health, this cause-and-effect relationship becomes very clear.

Researchers at Columbia University found eight major ways that toxins affect our health. They cause genomic mutations, epigenetic alterations, mitochondrial dysfunction, endocrine disruption, inflammation from oxidative stress; they also alter intercellular communication, interrupt microbiome communities, and impair nervous system function. We know that exposure to pollutants in air, water, soil, and food is harmful to human health. We are now learning about the specific biological pathways through which these chemicals damage our bodies. It is also becoming clear that exposure to common chemicals can bring about serious illness, even at relatively modest concentrations.

And while everyone will benefit from the elimination of environmental toxins, some people are more susceptible than others to negative effects from exposure. Genetics play a role, as do preexisting conditions and age. About 40 percent of the population cannot clear heavy metals from their body very well and are more susceptible to developing dementia from exposure to lead, mercury, and aluminum. We become more susceptible to the effects of toxins when we have an existing illness or infection. The very young and the very old are also at higher risk, from the same exposure, than the rest of the population. This means that even when everyone under the same roof has the same exposures, those who are more susceptible may develop disease, while others may have only mild symptoms.

The home detox program supports anyone who wants to maintain or enhance their health and energy. For those who are particularly susceptible to harm from environmental toxins, such as children and the elderly, the program provides much-needed protection. And for those who are already immune compromised, chronically ill, or chemically sensitive, it provides a blueprint for making changes that support health. Removing toxic exposures will reduce the burden on your cells, DNA, and microbiome, and allow the body to heal itself naturally.

REAL LIFE HOME DETOX

TOXINS AND YOUR KIDNEY FUNCTION

I worked with a mother and young daughter who had been diagnosed with reduced kidney function. When I arrived at their home, I discovered many fragranced products: plug-in air fresheners, air-freshening sprays, incense, perfumes, fragranced deodorant and menstrual care products, scented laundry detergent and dryer sheets, scented dishwasher soap, scented hand soap, scented candles, and fragranced cleaning products. This was the first clue to the cause of their health issues. Fragranced products contain a long list of toxins that directly affect the kidneys.

We spent several hours removing the fragranced products from the family home. The curtains and carpets were permeated with chemicals. We ran the curtains through several rounds of washing with unscented laundry soap and hot water before they were clean. We called in a carpet cleaning company that used natural enzymes to remove the chemicals from the carpets. All the surfaces in the house were thoroughly washed, including the walls, to remove the layers of chemical residue created by years of emissions from fragranced products. The entire process took about a week, but it was well worth the effort. Kidney function improved in both mother and daughter.

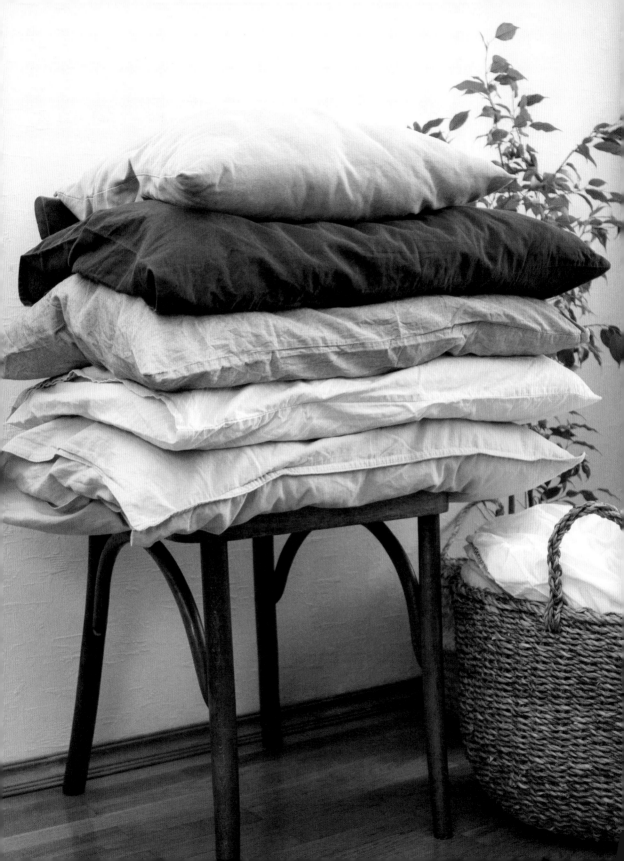

WHY ARE WE SURROUNDED BY TOXINS?

THE ANSWER LIES IN the fact that corporations have so much power and lack proper regulation of toxins in their products. Cleaning products are a good example. They comprise a multibillion-dollar-a-year industry with giant advertising budgets devoted to convincing us that we need these products for our convenience and safety. Ads are constantly pushing highly toxic products made by behemoth chemical companies, including Dow, DuPont, and Bayer. At the same time, there is inadequate government oversight of their claims and the safety of their products.

The laws governing labels on products are also weak. For example, acetaldehyde and benzene emit VOCs considered by the EPA to be carcinogenic and are unsafe at any exposure level. But because manufacturers aren't required to disclose a full list of ingredients on, for example, air freshener packaging, they often sneak these chemicals in under broader terms like "odor eliminator" or "fragrance." When you buy a household product, it's often impossible to know what you're purchasing unless you investigate each ingredient through a nongovernmental agency such as the Environmental Working Group.

The benefit in understanding our current system is that you will be better prepared to be a discerning shopper. When you're shopping for a household product, read the labels. Consider your options. Ask yourself: Is this product necessary? Do I know what its ingredients are? Are they safe to have in my home? If you can't answer yes to all of these criteria, don't buy it.

THE PATH FORWARD

CLEARLY, WE NEED SAFER OPTIONS. Most of us want to reduce our use of toxins, yet our society is not set up to make this possible without a tremendous amount of effort going into every decision we make throughout the day. We may want to use less plastic, for example, but it can be difficult to find something as simple as a toothbrush that's not made of plastic. It's hard to do the right thing for our bodies and the planet because we lack the infrastructure to help us.

That's where the home detox method can help. I've developed this system through decades of work helping people remove toxins and health threats from their homes. The work is grounded in evidence-based environmental health research. My intention in creating this simple method is to provide you with the best options for making your transformation to healthier living possible by removing toxins from your home and making cleaning simple and effective.

ABBREVIATIONS FOR CHEMICALS

Chemicals are in so many common household products and they are often abbreviated into acronyms, which further obscures them. Here is a handy list of many of the common chemicals present in our homes, along with their acronyms.

ACRONYMS FOR CHEMICAL COMPOUNDS

BFRs brominated flame retardants

BPA bisphenol A

BBP benzyl butyl phthalate

CO carbon monoxide

DBP dibutyl phthalate

DEA diethanolamine

DEG diethylene glycol

DEHP di(2-ethylhexyl) phthalate

DEGME diethylene glycol monomethyl ether

DINP diisononyl phthalate

EDC endocrine-disrupting chemical

EGME ethylene glycol monomethyl ether

HAP hazardous air pollutants

MEK methyl ethyl ketone

OPFRs organophosphate flame retardants

PDCB paradichlorobenzene

PFOA perfluorooctanoic acid

PBDE polybrominated diphenyl ether

PAH polycyclic aromatic hydrocarbon

PFAS polyfluoroalkyl substances

PTFE polytetrafluoroethylene

PVC polyvinyl chloride

SLS sodium lauryl sulfate

TCE trichloroethylene

TCC triclocarban

TCS triclosan

TEA triethanolamine

VOCs volatile organic compounds

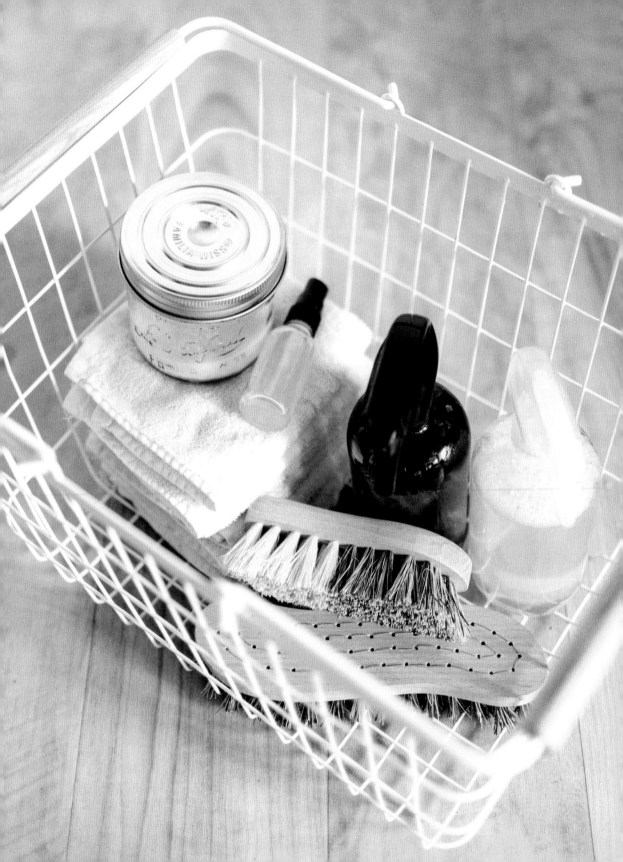

1

THE HOME DETOX METHOD

Detox cleaning is a method for removing pathogens and toxic residue on surfaces, in fabrics, and in the air. Let's go over the natural cleaning tools that can help you get each job done easily. I've included recipes for simple, natural cleaning solutions that effectively remove grease, grime, and harmful particulates. Some of these formulas, like Tub Scrub and Tea Tree Wash, are disinfectants that rely on proven antimicrobial ingredients, like tea tree essential oil, to eliminate viruses, fungi, and bacteria—without a single toxic ingredient. These homemade cleansers can replace the toxin-filled cleaning products you'll find at the grocery store.

CLEAN, NOT CHEMICAL

MOST COMMERCIAL cleaning products are full of highly caustic chemicals. Even the EPA notes that many common household cleaners contain VOCs, formaldehyde, and harsh acids. These products do damage to our bodies and the environment. Many of the degreasers used in these products, for example, can cause developmental, endocrine, reproductive, genetic, nervous system, and digestive system damage. When we stop to look at the research, it seems unfathomable that these products are legal. Until we have better governmental oversight for household products, we simply need to take matters into our own hands.

TOXINS IN OUR CLEANING PRODUCTS

Common commercial cleaning products are a significant source of toxins in our homes. Glass cleaners contain ethanolamine, isopropyl alcohol, and propylene glycol. Drain cleaners contain butoxyethanol, diethanolamine (DEA), sodium hydroxide, sodium hypochlorite (bleach), or triethanolamine (TEA). Surface cleaners contain butoxyethanol or diethylene glycol monomethyl ether (DEGME). Tile cleaners contain alcohol ethoxylates, alkylbenzene sulfonates, or sodium hypochlorite (bleach). Toilet cleaners contain ethanolamine, hydrofluoric acid, parabens, or propylene glycol. Avoiding these chemicals is one of the great benefits of making your own cleaning formulas at home.

CLEANING TOOLS

FIRST, LET'S REVIEW your cleaning tools, as they will be doing the bulk of the hard work for you. You may already have a few of the most helpful items, like scrub sponges, bristle brushes, and a vacuum that will filter the dust so that you aren't kicking it up into your lungs as you're cleaning. Use what you have and purchase the items you need so that your tools are ready when you begin your room-by-room home detox.

Air Purifiers

Air filtration is a game changer for those with allergies, autoimmune disease, or asthma. Air filters are also becoming popular in this era of forest fires and viruses as they can be effective tools for removing particulates (such as smoke or aerosol-borne viruses) from the air inside our homes. Portable air filters do a great job cleaning the air in a room where you spend a lot of time. I have units that not only filter but also cool or heat the air. During the fires that raged for months in my home state of Washington in 2020, I kept one unit in my bedroom and another in my office—the two rooms where I spend the most time—and kept them on around the clock.

Biodegradable Cleaning Gloves

If you're using nontoxic, food-grade cleaning solutions, gloves aren't necessary. But if you still would like your hands covered, opt for biodegradable or compostable gloves. Skip gloves made of vinyl, PVC, or synthetic latex.

Bottles and Jars

You'll need sturdy glass bottles and jars, with lids, in a variety of sizes and shapes for storing your homemade cleaning solutions. Canning jars are a good option; their glass is thick enough that they don't break easily, and the lids seal well. You can also simply reuse old peanut butter jars and the like, after cleaning them thoroughly and removing their labels. A short, widemouthed jar will work well for the Tub Scrub, and a tall, narrow bottle will do for the Liquid Laundry Soap.

Brooms

A well-made broom with properly cut fiber and a dustpan are must-haves. Bristles made of natural materials like bamboo, palm, straw, and vegetable fiber can last for generations, yet they are completely biodegradable and compostable. I particularly love the combination of design and function in the traditional natural-fiber brooms and brushes from Japan, Sweden, and Germany.

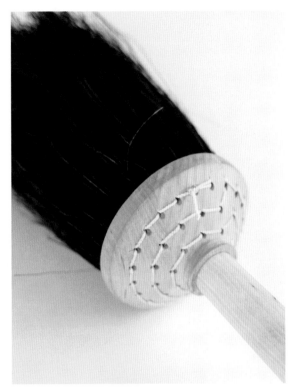

Look for a natural-fiber broom, such as this Swedish bassine outdoor broom made from palm leaves, which has just the right springiness so it sweeps well.

Dustpan

Look for a dustpan made of stainless steel, wood, bamboo, or some other natural material, rather than plastic. Match the size to the brush you will use with it. Think about how you will store it, too. If you want to hang it from a hook, look for a dustpan with a hole in its handle.

Cleaning Brushes

Brushes are critical. With the right brushes, you will find that you need very little cleaning solution—and you save some serious elbow grease. If you already own plastic scrub brushes, keep using them until they are

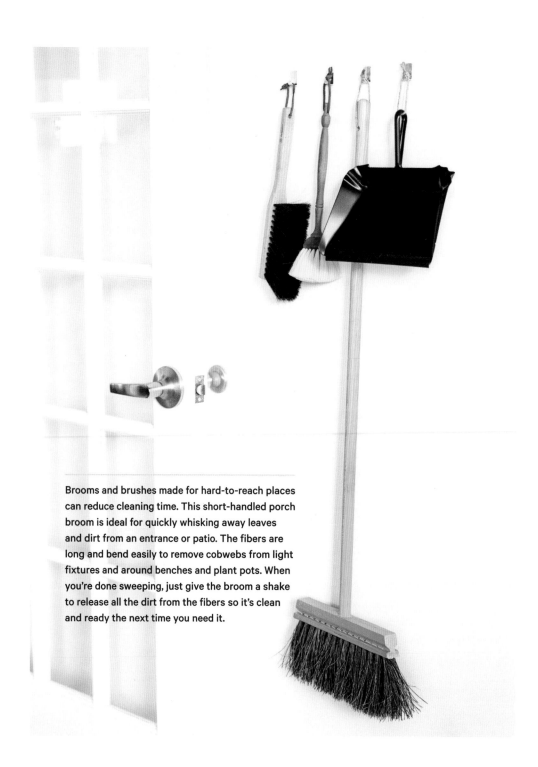

Brooms and brushes made for hard-to-reach places can reduce cleaning time. This short-handled porch broom is ideal for quickly whisking away leaves and dirt from an entrance or patio. The fibers are long and bend easily to remove cobwebs from light fixtures and around benches and plant pots. When you're done sweeping, just give the broom a shake to release all the dirt from the fibers so it's clean and ready the next time you need it.

completely worn out, rather than buying new brushes, to conserve resources. When you're ready to buy new cleaning brushes, look for wooden brushes with plant-based bristles.

Bucket or Caddy

A caddy or bucket that is easy to clean will work best. Look for a caddy that is large enough for all your cleaning gear, including scrub brushes, spray bottles, gloves, and vacuum attachments, and has a sturdy handle. If you have a small house, like I do, you can use one caddy to transport your supplies to each room as needed. If you have a large or multilevel home, you might choose to keep a caddy in each bathroom and one in the kitchen to save time.

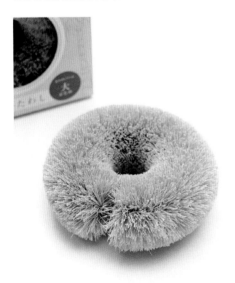

Tawashi cleaning brushes are durable. They make an excellent vegetable brush, and natural white palm fibers are good for heavy-duty pot scrubbing.

Rags

Old rags are good to have around for wiping up messes because you can toss them out guilt-free. Anything cotton that is at the end of its life can be made into rags. I cut up old towels and clothes and use socks like a glove when cleaning. I find that cotton cloth works better than paper towels; paper gets soggy and falls apart and you end up using a lot of it. Making paper towels requires industrial processing and many trees, so they are a real drain on our natural resources.

Microfiber cloths are popular, but microfiber is 80 percent polyester and 20 percent polyamide: plastic and chemicals! These cloths release microplastics into waterways and cannot be recycled or composted. Instead, look for cotton, hemp, and bamboo cloth rags, as they are biodegradable. I prefer 100 percent cotton terry cloth for cleaning and have a big stack of the washcloth size in my kitchen and cleaning caddy.

Retractable Razor Blade Scraper

You can use a sharp razor blade to scrape gunk from glass and other hard surfaces, saving yourself a great deal of scrubbing time and no chemical solvents are needed. When you're done, simply retract the blade back into its holder and then store it in your caddy so it's always with you as you are cleaning.

Sponges

Use sponges made of plant fibers like gourd, coconut shells, and walnut shells. They stay clean for a long time thanks to natural organic biocides that kill mold and bacteria. They are also eco-friendly because they're completely biodegradable. Avoid plastic sponges, as they contain phthalates and glues.

Spray Bottles

You'll want little spritzer bottles and larger spray bottles, preferably made of glass. Sprayer tops can be salvaged from empty product bottles and used for your own home-made solutions.

Vacuum

A proper vacuum cleaner is an essential tool for removing dust from nooks and crannies, and from carpet fibers. I prefer a vacuum with a washable filter rather than vacuum bags so that I don't have to keep vacuum bags on hand, plus it saves money and creates less waste. If you are sensitive to dust, look for a vacuum with a HEPA filter.

A natural-fiber rug beater is an excellent tool for cleaning rugs that are small enough to carry outside.

CLEANING UP AFTER PETS

We love our pets but let's face it, they make serious messes. I rely on two special tools to remove toxins created by pets. A black light can locate the mess, and enzymatic cleaners dissolve and remove the biological residue.

BLACK LIGHT. A black light urine detector is a flashlight that uses UV light to illuminate not only urine but also spray, feces, and barf residue on carpets and other surfaces. It can be incredibly helpful if you smell something funky and can't find the source. Turn off the lights and shine the black light over all surfaces to illuminate the source. Then you can target the site with some deep cleaning.

ENZYMATIC CLEANERS. Biological messes are protein based. Anywhere there are proteins, fungi and bacteria can grow, which means potential pathogens. Enzyme sprays are the most effective treatment for pet gunk. The enzymes break down the proteins so they can be completely removed.

MAKE YOUR OWN CLEANING SOLUTIONS

MAKING YOUR OWN cleaning solutions has three big advantages: no toxins, less expense, and less waste. By using ingredients like tea tree essential oil from a glass bottle, baking soda from a paper box, and real lemons, you skip all the chemicals and plastic packaging. This is important for our health and the planet, and these zero-waste solutions cost a small fraction of the bottled products found in most homes.

In my recipes for cleaning solutions, I rely on the following ingredients for their effectiveness, sustainability, low-waste packaging, and ease of access. Hopefully you can find everything you need at your local co-op or grocery store. Each ingredient has a purpose. Lemon juice and vinegar, for example, have acids that break down oily substances. Abrasives like baking soda and salt offer scrubbing ability. And antimicrobial essential oils kill bacteria, mold, and fungi.

One caveat about using essential oils: Remember that they are concentrated and powerful. They can be diluted in cleaning solutions, added to laundry water, or used full-strength in the soil around the house to deter pests. However, if drips of full-strength essential oils are left on paint or varnish, they can erode the surface. I learned this the hard way when a few drops landed on my new washing machine and left pockmarks.

Baking Soda

Baking soda, or sodium bicarbonate, is inexpensive and shelf stable for years. I use it in many of my cleaning solutions as a nontoxic abrasive.

Castile Bar Soap

Castile soap is any hard soap made from plant oils in a style similar to that originating in the Castile region of Spain. I use Dr. Bronner's Castile bar soap because the ingredients are clean and effective, and the company follows strict sustainability practices.

Essential Oils

Essential oils are volatile, aromatic oils extracted from plants. Many are potent antimicrobial agents.

My favorite antibacterial essential oils are eucalyptus, lemongrass, orange, palmarosa, patchouli, peppermint, and tea tree.

My favorite antifungal essential oils are citronella, geranium, lemongrass, orange, palmarosa, patchouli, and tea tree.

My top choice is tea tree essential oil because it is broadly antimicrobial, effective against bacteria, fungi (including mold), mildew, viruses, and mites, and it can be used in both cleaning solutions as well as personal care products like toothpaste and deodorant. I like the smell, too; it's so clean and earthy. Look for it in large bottles, which are, by the ounce, less expensive than the small bottles sold for cosmetic use.

When you're working with essential oils, look for organic, and always dilute them, as they are highly concentrated.

Grape Seed Extract

Grape seed extract, which has virtually no fragrance, is a potent antimicrobial agent. It can be used interchangeably for any essential oil in my cleaning recipes.

Sal Suds Liquid Cleaner

I use Dr. Bronner's Sal Suds Biodegradable Cleaner daily for dishes, laundry, floors, and other surfaces. Sal Suds is a concentrated all-purpose cleaner made with plant-based surfactants and natural fir needle and spruce essential oils without any synthetic dyes, fragrances, or preservatives. Sal Suds is concentrated and should be diluted with water. It lathers well and rinses out easily. It is also 100 percent cruelty-free, certified by the Coalition for Consumer Information on Cosmetics, and biodegrades rapidly.

Salt

Both table salt and coarse salt work well as gentle abrasives and are especially handy for jobs like scrubbing cast-iron pans.

Washing Soda

Washing soda, or sodium carbonate, softens water and helps lift soil from fabrics when used in combination with soap.

White Vinegar

Vinegar contains acetic acid produced by fermentation via bacteria. It bleaches, cuts grease, and breaks down minerals, such as lime buildup on faucets.

DO A PATCH TEST

Some fabrics and materials could be discolored or otherwise affected by cleaning solutions. The first time you use a new cleaning solution on any item of concern, test it on a small spot in an area that's not visible.

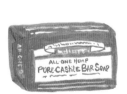
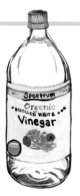
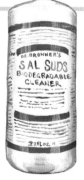
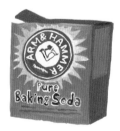
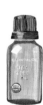

DETOX CLEANING SOLUTIONS

With a few simple ingredients, you can make all the household cleaning solutions you need. These are my go-to formulas; you may alter the recipes to meet your needs once you have tested them. For example, you might prefer to skip essential oils because the fragrance is too strong. Finding the right nontoxic solution for each cleaning task in your home should fit your personal preferences. Once you find the solutions you like, make a monthly ritual of preparing your solutions and organizing your tools. I like to make my solutions ahead of time so I can move through my cleaning chores easily.

· ● ·

DISHWASHER DETERGENT

Dishwasher detergent is often unnecessary. Dishwashers heat water to at least 140°F (60°C), the temperature needed to kill microbes. All you really need is a little baking soda to alkalize the water, which helps remove fats and proteins.

1 tablespoon baking soda

Pour the baking soda into the soap dispenser and run the dishwasher as usual.

· ● ·

DRAIN FIZZ

This works like a charm to unclog most slow bathroom and kitchen drains. Hot water melts away grease and soap residue, while the abrasive soda scrubs out and carries away any material lodged in the pipe. If baking soda and boiling water don't do the trick, add a few tablespoons of vinegar or lemon juice to help remove grease.

¼ cup baking soda
1 full teakettle of boiling water

Pour the baking soda directly into the drain and follow with the boiling water.

ESSENTIAL OIL SPRITZER

Water and essential oil are all you need to add fragrance to a room. If you're feeling creative, mix oils to create your own signature scent.

1 cup water
½ teaspoon essential oil (see page 15 for my favorites)

Combine the ingredients in a spray bottle, shake, and spritz as needed.

• ● •

FOAMING HAND SOAP

Foaming hand soap dispensers simply pull air into liquid soap so it comes out as foam. The beauty of this is that foam rinses away easily, less water is used, and diluting the soap conserves resources and money. Also, the dispensers can be reused and refilled. This light foam smells like pine trees.

1 cup water
1 tablespoon Dr. Bronner's Sal Suds

Combine water and Sal Suds in a foaming hand soap dispenser. Shake gently and pump.

• ● •

GLASS SPRAY

This simple cleaner works equally well for mirrors or windows. The acids in the vinegar help dissolve fingerprint oils and splatters on glass.

1 cup water
1 tablespoon white vinegar

Combine water and vinegar in a spray bottle. Spritz onto glass and wipe with a clean cotton cloth. Polish with a clean cloth until completely dry to avoid streaks.

LIQUID LAUNDRY SOAP

This works well for most fabrics and even shoes. One tablespoon of this liquid soap is enough for most loads of laundry. For heavily soiled laundry (with mold, grease, or grass stains), you may want to use 2 tablespoons. For unstained laundry like towels, sheets, and clothing, a teaspoon of undiluted Dr. Bronner's Sal Suds per load will do the job. The proportions here make a large batch, enough for 144 loads of laundry. I save my empty Sal Suds bottles and use them as dispensers.

7 cups water
1 cup Dr. Bronner's Sal Suds
1 cup washing soda

Bring the water to a boil in a large saucepan. Remove the pan from the heat. Add the Sal Suds and washing soda. Stir to dissolve. Let cool. Pour into jars or bottles.

• ● •

POWDERED LAUNDRY SOAP

Powdered soap works better than liquid for removing mud from fabric. However, some front-loading machines require liquid soap. Be sure to check your machine's instructions before adding powder to the soap receptacle. One tablespoon of this is enough for most laundry; you may need 2 or 3 tablespoons for large or extra-dirty loads.

1 cup grated Castile bar soap
1 cup baking soda
1 cup washing soda

Combine the grated soap, baking soda, and washing soda in a large bowl and mix well. Transfer to a storage container with an airtight lid; a large mason jar works well.

LIQUID DISH SOAP

Sal Suds is the best base for a liquid dish soap thanks to its ability to create bubbles and remove dirt and grease. A few full-strength drops right out of the bottle will go a long way and can be used for cleaning dishes, pans, and the sink. It can also be diluted, which will help it last longer and rinse easily. For disinfecting action as a safeguard against illness or to support immune-compromised household members, add a drop of tea tree essential oil.

1 cup Dr. Bronner's Sal Suds
1 cup water
1 drop tea tree essential oil (optional)

Combine Sal Suds and water in a dispenser or bottle and shake gently. Use as needed.

• ● •

PAN DEGREASER

This acidic combination breaks down fats and works well to remove grease buildup on pans and around stove hoods and vents. The solution will last a couple months in a cool, dark cupboard and longer in the refrigerator. The citrus juice residue can cause mold to develop in the lid of the jar, so I try to use up each batch within a few months.

A few citrus peels
2 cups white vinegar

Drop the citrus peels into a jar and add the vinegar, making sure that the peels are submerged in the liquid. Put on a lid and let the mixture sit for a few weeks so that the acidic vinegar can draw out the oils from the peels. Then remove the peels.

To use, apply a few tablespoons to a clean cloth or scrub sponge and wipe down greasy surfaces. Or pour the solution into a spray bottle, mist onto greasy surfaces, and wipe with a dry cloth.

TEA TREE WASH

This sudsy formula will clean and disinfect any surface, including walls, floors, carpets, countertops, toilets, sinks, and toys.

2 cups water
1 tablespoon Dr. Bronner's Sal Suds
1 tablespoon tea tree essential oil
Few drops of essential oil for fragrance (optional)

Combine the water, Sal Suds, tea tree oil, and a few drops of essential oil of your choice for fragrance (if desired) in a spray bottle. When you're ready to use it, give the bottle a shake to mix the contents and spray it on surfaces. Let it sit for a minute to kill microorganisms and then wipe away with a clean damp cloth.

• ● •

TUB SCRUB

This scrubby stuff works wonders on porcelain. It's also effective for cleaning ovens and any surface that requires some scrubbing action, all while disinfecting and smelling great. Use a large scrub brush for tubs and a vegetable fiber sponge for pans. You can adjust the water-to-soda ratio as needed; more baking soda will give you a thicker mixture for ovens, and more water will provide easier coverage on large surfaces like vinyl floors.

1 cup water
1 cup baking soda
1 tablespoon Dr. Bronner's Sal Suds
1 teaspoon tea tree essential oil

Combine the water, baking soda, Sal Suds, and tea tree oil in a wide-mouthed jar and mix well.

To use, scoop out a few tablespoons, and use a cloth to apply the thin paste to surfaces. Scrub gently, then wipe clean with a dry cloth.

IDENTIFYING THE TOXIC TEN

AS PART OF YOUR HOME DETOX, you will learn the top ten toxins in each room. Then you will target these highly toxic items and remove, replace, or modify them. Some of these items can be recycled or tossed out, while others will need to be replaced. Before you bring new items into your home, think about whether they are necessary. We don't really need much to function efficiently, and the more we can do without, the less risk we have for toxins, not to mention cluttered shelves and expense. When you do purchase new items, read labels carefully and only buy those that are completely nontoxic.

Supertoxins

A few items are so dangerous that I call them *supertoxins*. These items emit such high levels of chemicals into the air that once we've breathed them in and absorbed them into our bloodstream, they can cause a host of debilitating health conditions. They are the cause of a wide range of symptoms of poor health, such as asthma, headaches, inflammation, and fatigue. As a first step, I generally ask my clients to remove these items from their homes and then monitor their health to see if their symptoms improve, and they often report a positive effect in a short time.

AIR FRESHENERS. Commercial spray products, plug-ins, candles, fragrant oil warmers, and even the tree-shaped hanging car air fresheners emit a host of seriously toxic chemicals, including solvents and formaldehyde.

BROMINATED FLAME RETARDANTS. Brominated flame retardants (BFRs) are used in many consumer products, including fabrics and plastics. These products release BFRs when they become heated, for example by an electrical current in kitchen appliances and TVs, or from body heat in crib mattresses and clothing.

TEFLON AND OTHER FLUOROPOLYMERS. Many nonstick pans are coated with fluoropolymers like polytetrafluoroethylene (the best known is Teflon). Toxic chemical compounds found in these polymers can become airborne when the pans are heated, especially at high temperatures. When the nonstick coating is scratched, it can release toxic particles into the food we are cooking, and we end up ingesting them.

BATH BOMBS. These balls of chemicals disintegrate in water, releasing VOCs and solvents into bathwater and into the enclosed air of the bathroom, and we then absorb them through our skin and lungs.

DRYER SHEETS. As these chemical sheets heat up in the dryer, their solvents, synthetic fragrances, and VOCs are released into the air inside the home and also blown out the dryer vent into the air around the home, exposing both humans and animals to highly active compounds that carry health risks.

INCENSE. When we burn incense, VOCs and solvents are released that can be detected by their odor throughout the house and the smoke that settles on surfaces. The chemicals remain active on clothing, bedding, curtains, and other household fabrics, continuing to expose people and pets to health risks.

MEMORY FOAM. Memory foam contains mostly polyurethane, which off-gases, filling the air with VOCs, heavy metals, and toxic acids, ethers, and solvents. Sleeping on synthetic memory foam night after night dramatically increases the level of exposure.

REDUCE WASTE

Landfills across the United States are full, and many other countries are no longer accepting our refuse. Many recycling centers are so overloaded that they are no longer accepting new materials. So even when we buy something that is technically considered recyclable, it may still end up in a landfill at the end of its life, further burdening our environment.

DETOX CLEANING

I provide a **Detox Clean** section for every room—a guide to residual and hidden toxins that need to be properly "detox cleaned." These areas generally need greater focus and attention to clean out the dust, microbes, and chemicals. Grab your cleaning caddy with your tools and cleaning solutions and work your way through the area. After that first effort, the whole house can be easily maintained with lighter weekly cleanings.

You now have what you need to take on the role of toxin detective, searching out and removing toxins from your home. Take it one step at a time, room by room.

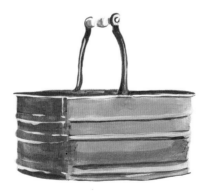

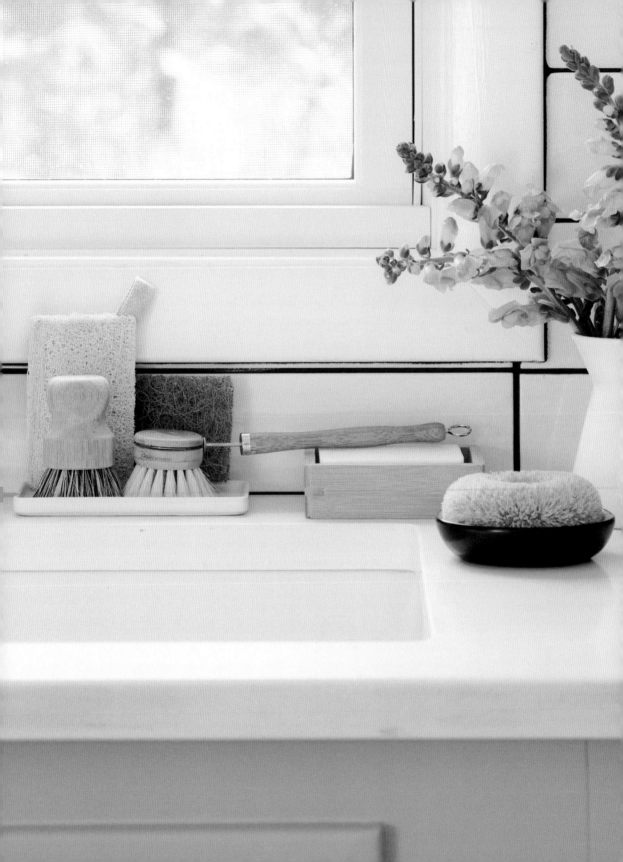

2
KITCHEN

Kitchens play an important role in supporting our well-being, but the average kitchen is a bit of a minefield, with toxins in food packaging, cooking equipment, utensils, and other items. In terms of detoxification, the kitchen is the most critical room in the home because so many kitchen toxins touch our food and water. While in the rest of the house we are exposed to toxins primarily through our lungs and skin, here we also have the potential for ingestion. Let's start our room-by-room detox program here in the kitchen, which for many of us is the central hub of the household.

HIDDEN TOXINS IN THE KITCHEN

IT'S EASY TO FIND TOXINS in your kitchen if you know what to look for. As you work your way through the kitchen, you may need to replace some items you rely on, but nontoxic alternatives can be found. For example, nonstick ceramic pans in place of Teflon, beeswax food wrap in place of plastic, and glass food storage containers with cork lids in place of plastic. Once you have removed all the sources of toxins, deep cleaned, and wiped away dust and residue, you can relax, knowing you have created a truly toxin-free kitchen.

Aluminum

Aluminum is a heavy metal that acts as a neurotoxin and has been linked to anemia, encephalopathy, multiple sclerosis, dementia, Alzheimer's disease, and breast cancer. Even with this information, it is still being used in products that touch our food. It is, for example, used in foil, pie pans, cans, aseptic packaging, cookware, and utensils from cheese graters to spatulas, and they all leach this heavy metal into our food. Processed foods are highly contaminated by aluminum due to its use in manufacturing facilities and packaging.

As you look through your kitchen for aluminum to eliminate, consider some swaps. Aluminum foil is often used as a lid when baking. Instead, use a baking dish with its own lid, such as a Dutch oven or a crockpot. If you have aluminum baking sheets, switch to stainless steel or use a layer of parchment paper as a barrier between your food and the baking sheets. Replace aluminum pans with stainless steel, cast iron, copper, or ceramic.

Note that many pans have an aluminum core under an outer layer of another material, like stainless steel. The aluminum core is used to keep the pans lightweight. In this case, the aluminum does not come in contact with food, so these pans are nontoxic.

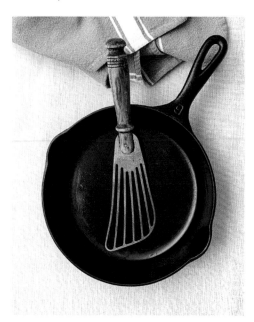

Well-seasoned cast-iron cookware is easy to clean, long-lasting, nontoxic, and inexpensive.

TOXIC TEN

1. ALUMINUM
2. COFFEE PODS
3. CUTTING BOARDS
4. FOOD PACKAGING
5. FOOD STORAGE CONTAINERS
6. SOAP
7. SPONGES
8. TAP WATER
9. TEFLON AND NONSTICK COOKWARE
10. UTENSILS

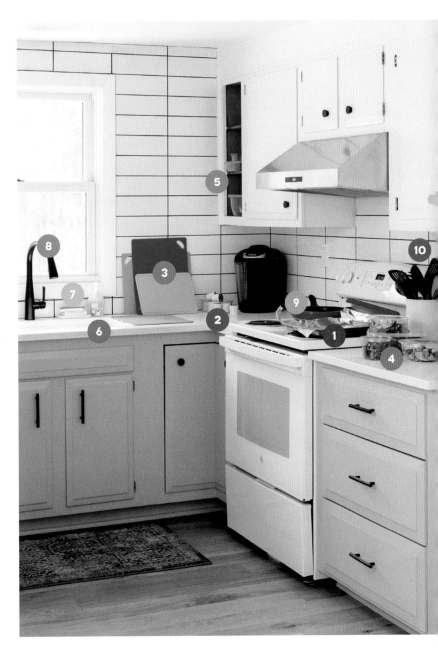

ALUMINUM AND CANCER MARKERS

I worked with a woman who had metastatic breast cancer. I ran several tests for well-known breast cancer toxins, including plastics, metals, and parabens. In her case, we found only one suspect, aluminum, which was significantly elevated in her urine. With this clue, we went through her kitchen looking for culprits and found many old aluminum kitchen tools, including pans and utensils, which had been her mother's. She used them often, and they were likely the source of contamination. I suggested she get rid of them. Rather than tossing them, she decided to put them on display in a glass cabinet with her old dish sets so she could hold on to the memories but not use them for cooking.

After six weeks of supplements to support her body's ability to excrete metals, her urine was clear of aluminum. Soon after, we learned that her cancer markers (the numbers oncologists use to monitor cancer cells) had gone down significantly. I have been testing clients for toxins for decades now, and it is always thrilling to see such fast improvement with relatively little effort.

Coffee Pods

The first time I saw a coffee pod machine, I yelled "Noooo!" right there in the store. It was obvious that this system of single-use plastic cups was being marketed as the trendy new way to make gourmet coffee at home, and it was only a matter of time before these toxic time-saver pods would be floating up on our beaches and adding to our phthalate-driven diseases.

Coffee pods have become so popular that now more than 24 million are used each day! When hot water is forced through these single-use plastic cups, the heat carries high levels of phthalates and other chemicals into the cup of brew—and then we drink it. The pods are a disaster for human health and the planet.

Recently, manufacturers have started using recycled plastic to make the pods. This sounds like a good idea, but recycled plastics have a high toxic load of formaldehyde due to the way that various types of plastics are melded together at recycling centers. The level of contamination is so high that formaldehyde is now detectable in the coffee that is made from these recycled pods.

It might shock you to learn that all coffee brewed from these pods contains appreciable amounts of lead and nickel. Daily exposure to the heavy metals and phthalates leaching from the pods can accumulate to levels that cause hormonal changes, breast cancer development, hardening of the arteries, dementia, and autoimmune conditions.

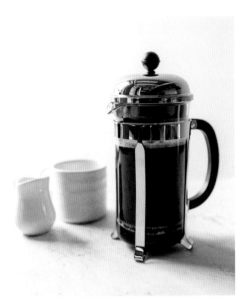

A French press made of glass and stainless steel is a nontoxic alternative to plastic coffee makers.

There are many good alternatives to coffee pods. For example, pour-over brewing with a stainless-steel dripper is nontoxic and doesn't even require a paper filter. If you're making coffee for more than one person, using a glass French press is a quick and simple method, and it comes in many sizes.

Cutting Boards

We use cutting boards constantly when we're eating healthy because eating healthy means vegetables, and vegetables mean a whole lot of chopping. Those cutting boards really are the heart of the kitchen. Anything we use daily is a critical item to scrutinize for toxins, and the culprit here is plastic cutting boards. The plastic is so soft that when knives cut through food, they also cut into the boards, chopping little slices of plastic and potentially

phthalates into our food. This is one of the reasons we end up ingesting a credit card's worth of plastic every week!

Beyond the phthalates from plastics, many plastic cutting boards harbor another synthetic chemical: a triclosan treatment used to kill bacteria. Triclosan has been linked to cancer, immune suppression, and diabetes due to its effect on the microbial ecosystem in our bodies. Studies have found it to be an endocrine toxin. The FDA itself issued a warning based on studies showing that exposure to high doses of triclosan is associated with decreased levels of thyroid hormones in animals.

As an alternative to plastic, I like hardwood, bamboo, or pressed paper cutting boards because they are nontoxic and durable. Marble is another option; it is impermeable to microbes, but it's so heavy that it will likely get only a cursory wipe-down rather than being run through the dishwasher or scrubbed properly in the sink. Also, hard surfaces like marble will dull your knives.

Choose cutting boards for daily use that are large enough to give you plenty of working space, but not so large they won't fit in the sink or dishwasher for cleaning. I prefer to sterilize my cutting boards by running them through the dishwasher. I do so daily, even with my pressed-paper boards, and they have stayed in great shape, so there's no need to worry about damaging them by overwashing. If you don't have a dishwasher, or if you have wooden cutting boards that can't go in the dishwasher, you can sterilize them with tea tree essential oil. Spray Tea Tree Wash (page 21) on a board, let it sit for about 10 minutes, then rinse well.

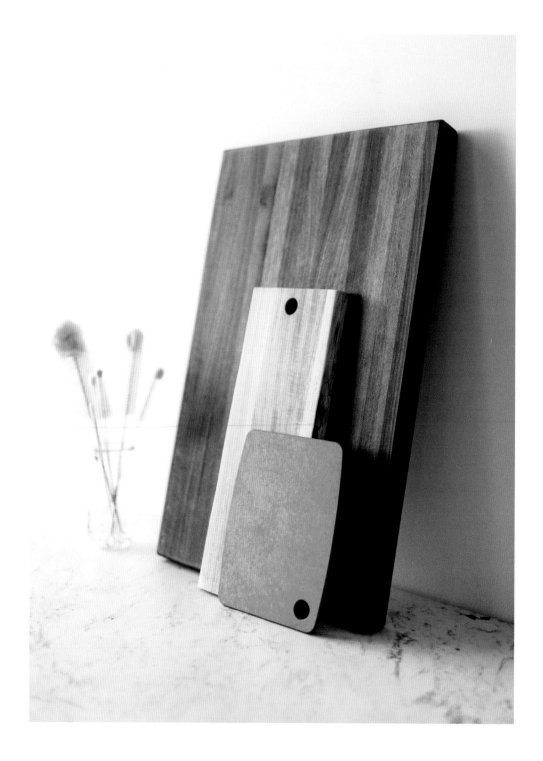

RECYCLED PLASTIC AND FLAME RETARDANTS

When plastics that contain flame retardants are recycled to make new products, they can carry those toxins to the new products. Brominated flame retardants (BFRs) are supertoxins that have been linked to thyroid disease and cancer. They are so dangerous to human health that some BFRs are no longer allowed in the manufacturing of new products. However, when old items that contain BFRs are recycled and then used to make new items, the new items can contain BFRs. That can be the case for kitchen gear made from recycled plastic, like cutting boards and kitchen utensils. It's why many of the inexpensive black plastic utensils test high for BFRs—and it's one more good reason to steer clear of plastic in the kitchen.

WOODEN CUTTING BOARDS NEED EXTRA CARE. Wooden cutting boards are more prone to microbial growth than those made from denser materials like pressed paper. They require frequent scrubbing with something gritty, like baking soda or coarse salt, to draw out and remove some of the microbes that linger in wood and create odors. When wooden boards are used heavily, the surface gets roughed up and becomes porous, so that it may not dry well between uses. Then it becomes an ever-moist place where bacteria and fungi grow easily. The only way to save a wooden board at this point is to sand the surface down smooth again. Your boards may also benefit from a light rubbing of vegetable oil to protect the wood from drying out and cracking. This can be done with a clean cloth and a teaspoon of vegetable oil.

Food Packaging

Each year, 174 million tons of plastic food packaging is produced globally. Packaged food is known for being unhealthy due to its lack of nutrients; and just as concerning as the low-quality processed foods they contain is the concern for the high levels of toxins from the food containers themselves. Styrofoam (polystyrene) food containers leach styrene and benzene into food; both are suspected carcinogens and known neurotoxins. Plastic containers release bisphenols and phthalates into foods. Even plastics that are BPA-free may contain other types of bisphenols.

Most packaged foods sold in grocery stores are in containers made of plastic. Even products that at first glance look innocuous, like paper cups and milk cartons, are usually lined with plastic to make them waterproof, and metal cans are lined with plastic to prevent rust. This packaging is a significant source of the plastic particles (and chemicals from plastic) that we ingest.

Long-term chronic exposure to, and ingestion of, plastic carries a high risk of triggering health problems. Illnesses linked to plastic exposure include atherosclerosis, autoimmune disease, breast cancer, diabetes, heart disease, hormonal imbalances, infertility, polycystic ovary syndrome, and prostate cancer.

The deluge of plastic—in containers, packaging, toys, tools, home goods, and more—is part of a greater problem. We have so much plastic in the world that it's found in micro- and nanoparticles everywhere: in our blood, our water supply, and even the rain. This is why, now more than ever, we need to stand up and say no to plastics!

AVOID PLASTIC PACKAGING. We can protect ourselves and our planet by making small changes in our habits. Skip the strawberries and lettuce sold in plastic clamshells. Buy whole, unpackaged foods from the produce and bulk sections of the grocery store. Avoid the plastic bags available in the produce section by bringing reusable cloth or cotton mesh bags. Buy spices, grains, legumes, and any other item you can in bulk and store them in glass jars.

Purchasing directly from local farmers is a great way to support your health and the environment. The nonprofit Local Harvest offers a simple online search engine that can help you find farms, farmers' markets, farm stands, and community-supported agriculture (CSA) programs in your area. Eating locally leads to eating seasonally, which means your food will be as nutrient-rich as it can be by coming freshly harvested to your plate.

If you do buy packaged foods, minimize the plastic packaging. For example, you could buy pasta in a plastic bag, but a pasta box is only about 20 percent plastic, and the rest is cardboard, making the box a better option. As a general rule for grocery shopping, a

company that sells its food in environmentally hazardous packaging isn't worth your dollar. We have a huge (plastic) mountain to climb, but our choices will affect the evolution of industry, and voting with our dollars will reduce the production of plastic packaging, our exposure, and waste.

Plastic toxins are more likely to migrate into food that is hot, wet, or acidic, so do your best to avoid these situations. Never microwave or otherwise heat food in plastic; it expedites leaching.

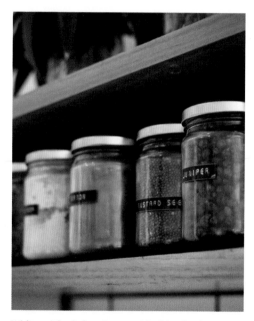

Widemouthed glass jars are ideal for food storage. Save your jars and remove the labels so you can easily see what you have stored inside them.

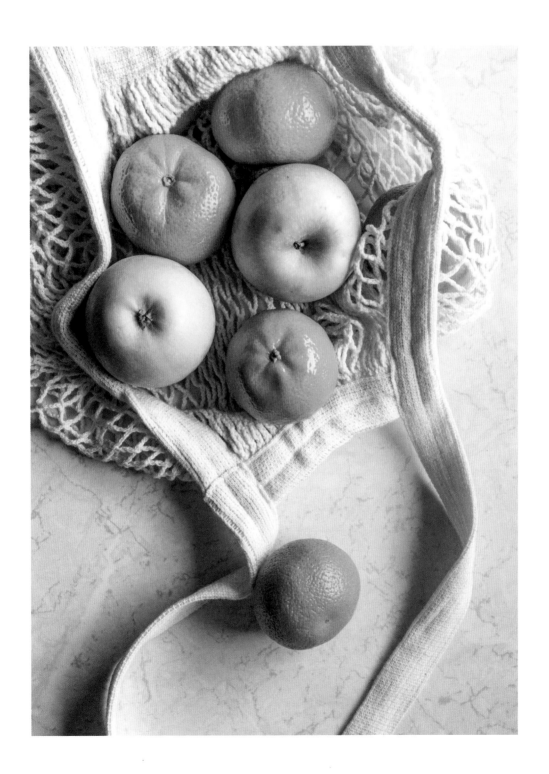

Food Storage Containers

Around the world, we use millions of rolls of plastic wrap each year for food storage. This wrapping leaches toxins into food. Fortunately, after decades of plastic wrap, ziplock bags, and plastic containers, our food storage options are finally changing. We are now seeing more biodegradable alternatives to plastic, such as paper, bioplastics, and mushroom-based packaging, and they continue to evolve in the right direction for our health, sustainability, and durability.

It's best to avoid plastic for food storage. At home, replace your plastic storage containers with glass, and use lids that are stainless steel, cork, or wood. Glass jars also work well for storing food and beverages. Canning jars are low cost and can be purchased at hardware stores. I use widemouthed glass canning jars; they're durable, the rubber around the rim is biodegradable, and they come in large sizes, which allows me to store premade meals to take on the road and eat right out of the jar. But you don't have to run out and buy a whole set of new containers. Some of my favorite jars are the ones I save and reuse from foods like jam, olives, peanut butter, and tomato sauce.

REAL LIFE HOME DETOX

PCOS AND PLASTIC

I learned how challenging it can be to identify sources of plastic toxins while making a house call to consult with a young woman with polycystic ovary syndrome (PCOS). PCOS is the most common endocrine disease among reproductive-aged women in the United States. It's a complex condition that often overlaps with hormonal imbalances, metabolic syndromes, and insulin resistance. Phthalates from plastics are a primary trigger for PCOS as they are powerful endocrine disruptors that mimic hormones and throw off healthy hormone levels.

We had been working together for months on the phone, discussing how plastic releases phthalates that drive PCOS. She had reported that she was no longer eating out of plastic or microwaving in plastic. Upon entering her home, I became aware that my client didn't understand which items in her home contained plastic. There were Starbucks cardboard cups on the counter, which are lined with plastic and have plastic lids that touch the hot liquid as we drink it. I looked in the refrigerator and pulled out dozens of plastic produce bags and cardboard containers of milk and juice that are also lined with plastic. I also spotted plastic wrappers from snack foods and plastic to-go boxes from restaurants. This was a horror scene for a nutritionist! Each of these items posed a significant risk for this young woman. My client had plastics flooding her kitchen, and she really wasn't seeing it.

Silicone bags and jar lids are more environmentally friendly than plastic in that they aren't toxic and can be reused. However, silicone is not biodegradable and will end up in the landfill eventually.

You can replace plastic wrap with beeswax wraps. These beeswax-coated cloths work well for wrapping up sandwiches, covering bowls, and so on. They can be washed and reused many times, and they're completely nontoxic and biodegradable. Waxed paper is another option for wrapping up food; just be sure to buy a natural brand because some commercial brands may contain nonstick chemicals such as polytetrafluoroethylene (PTFE).

HIDDEN IN PLAIN SIGHT. When I point out plastic sources to my friends and clients, they are always a little freaked out to discover that plastic was there all along, but it was invisible to them. Plastics have become such an integral part of our lives that we must practice extreme vigilance to avoid them. I have been passionate about this work for years now, but at the end of the day I still look around and see where plastic has slipped in. Plastic is in the packages I order online, the pots holding my houseplants, and the lining of the cans of my cat's food. The process of change requires small steps in the right direction. Recently, I made the decision to stop ordering from certain major companies because of their plastic shipping material. I decided to investigate the eco-friendly online companies I order from to make sure they use completely biodegradable packaging. I talked with my local garden store about taking back my plastic plant pots to reuse. I am also making my cat's meals from whole foods to avoid pet food cans altogether.

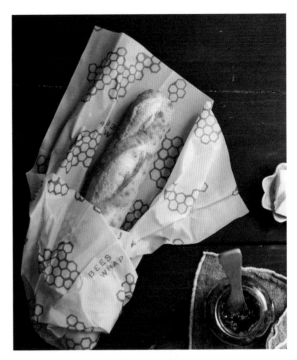

Beeswax wrap is made from organic cotton, beeswax, jojoba oil, and tree resin, and is washable, reusable, and compostable.

Soap

Many antibacterial soaps contain triclosan. This chemical is added to products for its antimicrobial effect, but it weakens the immune system, according to studies performed by the National Institutes of Heath (NIH), Centers for Disease Control and Prevention (CDC), and dozens of other independent sources. There is also evidence to suggest that children exposed to triclosan at an early age have an increased chance of developing allergies, asthma, and eczema. Triclosan alters gut microbiota, which has a pro-inflammatory effect, especially in the digestive tract, and is now linked to digestive issues, diabetes, and other blood sugar disorders. Even infrequent exposures can cause low-grade colonic inflammation and exacerbate colitis-associated colon cancer. This synthetic antiseptic is dangerous and unnecessary. Use good old-fashioned soap instead, which has been shown to be as effective as, if not more effective than, triclosan in real-world situations.

Another consideration is fragrance in hand and dish soaps. Volatile organic compounds (VOCs) from synthetic fragrances act as free radicals, irritating tissues, triggering inflammation, and even bringing on asthma attacks. Fragrances in soaps trigger migraines for many people. Look for unscented soap products.

Our skin contains many bacteria that are beneficial to our health. Using natural soap and hot water will leave the symbiotic, healthy microbes in skin, while removing viruses and bad bacteria from the surface. Grape seed extract and tea tree essential oil are both highly effective antimicrobials that can be added to liquid soap as an extra protection. However, viruses are eradicated simply by washing hands with soap and hot water for two minutes. Look for soaps that are vegan, biodegradable, and free of sulfates, parabens, synthetic fragrances, and palm oil.

Sponges

Plastic dish sponges should be a thing of the past. They release bits of plastic and dyes into the water system, and eventually these toxins end up downstream, harming ocean life. They can also harbor high levels of *Acinetobacter*, bacteria that can cause upper and lower respiratory tract infections, inner ear inflammation, pinkeye, inflammation of the cornea of the eye, and sinusitis.

Thanks to eco-conscious companies, natural sponges are more accessible than ever. Plant-fiber sponges clean fruits and veggies well, are strong enough for the greasy jobs, and don't scratch pans. Plant-based sponges dry easily, too, which means less moisture in which bacteria can grow, and they are compostable and biodegradable.

Tap Water

Clean water is getting harder to come by due in large part to environmental pollution. Water that flows from the taps in our homes can be contaminated with chemicals, heavy metals, and pathogens, and often is. Water from open aquifers is affected by air pollution, water from wells is exposed to anything in the local water table (industrial or natural environmental contaminants), and water held in metal cisterns may carry mold and leached metals. When water leaves its holding area and heads to your home, it runs through pipes that may contain lead or are made of polyvinyl chloride (PVC). Lead water pipes, which were in use until the 1970s, when they were banned, leach lead into tap water. Older homes and municipalities with older water systems may still have this problem. Today, lead solder is still sometimes used to connect and repair water pipes. Keep in mind that even low levels of exposure to lead can affect memory and cause learning disabilities as well as behavioral problems. Higher levels of exposure and sustained or repeated exposure can lead to neurological problems, amyotrophic lateral sclerosis (ALS, or Lou Gehrig's disease), kidney damage, high blood pressure, disrupted blood cell production, and reproductive problems.

Some pollution that affects our water starts in our own homes. For example, the residue of many popular medications, like birth control pills, statin drugs, nonsteroidal anti-inflammatories (ibuprofen), and antidepressants, contaminate our drinking water and the environment. We pee out a substantial amount of the drugs we take in. Researchers recently tested drinking water from more than a thousand aquifers across the United States and found 21 hormones and 103 pharmaceuticals in most of the samples. Another study found bisphenol A, high levels of three pharmaceutical drugs, and a caffeine by-product in tap water samples.

Herbicides and pesticides are a significant source of heavy metal contamination of ground water. In some areas of the world, drinking-water sources have been highly contaminated with arsenic, exposing an estimated 160 million people to levels that increase the incidence of lung cancer.

Fluoride in our drinking water is another problem. A study published by Mount Sinai researchers found that fluoride exposure can lead to a reduction in kidney and liver function among children and adolescents. At the same time, children's exposure to fluoride is increasing due to the artificial fluoridation of municipal water in many cities. Municipalities treat their water with fluoride because fluoride prevents tooth decay. Tooth decay is a nationwide issue due to the standard American diet, which is high in sugar. Dietary sugar feeds the bacteria that cause tooth decay. So, the root of the problem is too much sugar. Despite the proven

risk that fluoride carries for human health, the CDC still encourages the practice of fluoridation, which is a powerful example of how our society lacks the science-based regulation we need to protect us from toxins, and why it is so critical that we take matters into our own hands to protect ourselves and our families.

Bottled water is not the answer, as it is a common source of plastic toxins. According to a recent study's findings, 93 percent of bottled water showed signs of microplastic contamination.

The takeaway is that we must filter the water in our homes until these issues are resolved. Look for solid carbon filters or reverse-osmosis systems, which remove common contaminants, including agricultural chemicals, heavy metals, microplastics, fluoride, decaying organic matter, and medications.

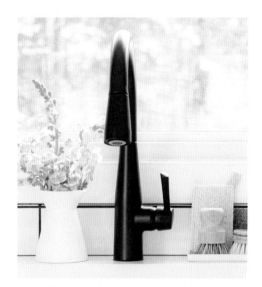

Water filtration units can be attached directly to the kitchen faucet or installed under the sink and out of the way.

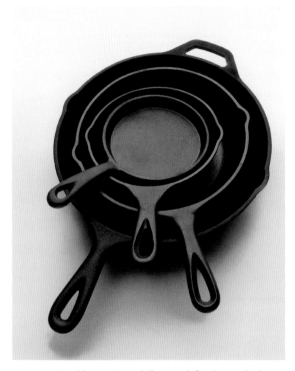

Durable cast-iron skillets cook foods evenly due to their thermal density.

Teflon and Fluoropolymer Nonstick Coatings

Many of the pots, pans, baking sheets, rice cookers, and other equipment we use in the kitchen have nonstick coatings made of fluoropolymers, a type of fluorocarbon-based resin. These polymers are used to make products resistant to stains, grease, and water and to reduce friction—that is, to make them nonstick. The most well known is Teflon, which is, technically, polytetrafluoroethylene (PTFE).

While a nonstick surface certainly makes cooking easier, this convenience comes with a cost. Fluoropolymers belong to a group of highly toxic compounds known as per- and polyfluoroalkyl substances (PFAS). PFAS are associated with a wide array of diseases, including endocrine, kidney, and thyroid disruption, elevated cholesterol levels, developmental issues, metabolic changes, and cancer. Breast tissue is particularly vulnerable; PFAS are considered carcinogenic mammary toxicants.

While PFAS have many applications and are used in many products, they are especially dangerous in our cookware. When a Teflon pan gets scratched, it releases particles of PTFE into the food we are cooking, and we end up ingesting them. Also, when PFAS are heated to high temperatures, they can off-gas noxious chemicals, which we then breathe.

I recommend immediately removing from your home any nonstick cookware that uses PFAS. There are some wonderful nontoxic alternatives, including seasoned cast iron, stainless steel, and ceramic nonstick. Buy the highest-quality pans you can afford; they will keep you safe and will last for generations if well cared for.

Once you have invested in nontoxic cookware, you can protect ceramic nonstick surfaces by avoiding metal utensils, which can damage them. The best options are utensils made from wood, bamboo, or silicone, which are all soft enough that they won't scratch. Cast-iron cookware is an exception; it is scratch resistant, and you can use even stainless-steel utensils with it.

Utensils

Cooking utensils can contain a variety of toxins. Many, and especially the black nylon type, contain diamino diphenylmethane (DDM), an epoxy hardener. When we use utensils at high heat, they can melt, releasing DDM into our food.

TEFLON FLU

I saw the effects of "Teflon flu" firsthand with a client who started having breathing problems and a dry cough. A chest scan showed inflammation in both lungs. I made a home visit to try to help him identify possible triggers for this sudden inflammation. We started in the kitchen, and I saw the culprit right away: a visibly scratched and peeling Teflon pan. I suggested that his respiratory inflammation could be from exposure to the toxic gases released from his Teflon pan. The blackened bottom of the pan made me realize he was also using high heat when cooking. This combination causes high levels of PFA gases, which when inhaled can trigger lung inflammation that can lead to polymer fume fever, also known as Teflon flu.

My client replaced the pan with a cast-iron skillet and started ventilating the area by opening windows when he cooked. These few steps were enough to help his symptoms subside, and his lungs were again functioning normally within about a week after he took action.

DDM is listed as a known carcinogen by the CDC and is known to cause cirrhosis and tumors.

Formaldehyde is another common toxin found in utensils. Melamine dishware, such as plates, cups, and utensils, are made with formaldehyde. If melamine items get too hot, they can melt and leach chemicals into food and drinks. One study of melamine cookware showed the migration of formaldehyde from the cookware into food in seven of the ten samples tested.

Also, many plastic utensils are now made from recycled plastics that contain brominated flame retardants (BFRs).

Nylon and plastic utensils aren't a risk worth taking in your kitchen. Nontoxic alternatives include stainless steel, silicone, bamboo, and wood.

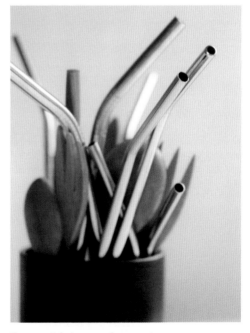

Onyx metal straws reduce waste.

Hidden Toxins in the Kitchen

KIDNEY TOXINS

Chronic kidney disease affects at least one in seven Americans and 10 percent of the world population. By understanding that toxins play a significant role in kidney disease, you can take action to reduce your risk of or even reverse this debilitating illness.

This chart lists toxins that affect kidneys and examples of common sources. It is by no means complete. There are thousands of toxins in the home that stress the kidneys. The toxins that we ingest, absorb, and inhale are filtered through the kidneys and ultimately excreted through the urinary tract. It's no surprise that kidney issues are on the rise as levels of environmental pollutants increase.

KIDNEY TOXINS AND THEIR HOUSEHOLD SOURCES

acetaldehyde synthetic carpets, dryer sheets

acetone nail polish remover, dryer sheets

antimony trioxide memory foam

arsenic tap water, pressure-treated wood

benzene dryer sheets

bromine dough conditioners, flame retardants, pool disinfectant

carbon monoxide gas leaks, candles

diethylene glycol air fresheners

diisocyanates polyurethane foam insulation

ethanol dryer sheets

ethyl acetate nail polish, nail polish remover

ethylene glycol windshield fluid

fluoride toothpaste, mouthwash, teeth whitening strips

haloacetic acid chlorinated tap water

hydramethylnon roach killer

lead children's toys, mini blinds, car batteries

naphthalene mothballs

paradichlorobenzene mothballs

PBDE memory foam, plastic

PFA nonstick pans, stain-resistant fabrics, waterproofing spray, dental floss, stain-resistant carpet, glues

PTFE dental floss, nonstick cookware

terpene laminate wood

toluene composite wood, cigarette smoke, nail polish, nail polish remover, synthetic fragrances, paint thinners, glue

trichloroethylene paint remover, degreasers

VOC incense, perfumes, plastics, dryer sheets, scented candles, memory foam, fragranced products, synthetic latex, glues, varnishes, polyurethane foam, paint thinners

xylene paint, lacquer, adhesives, rust preventers, paint thinners, gasoline, permanent markers

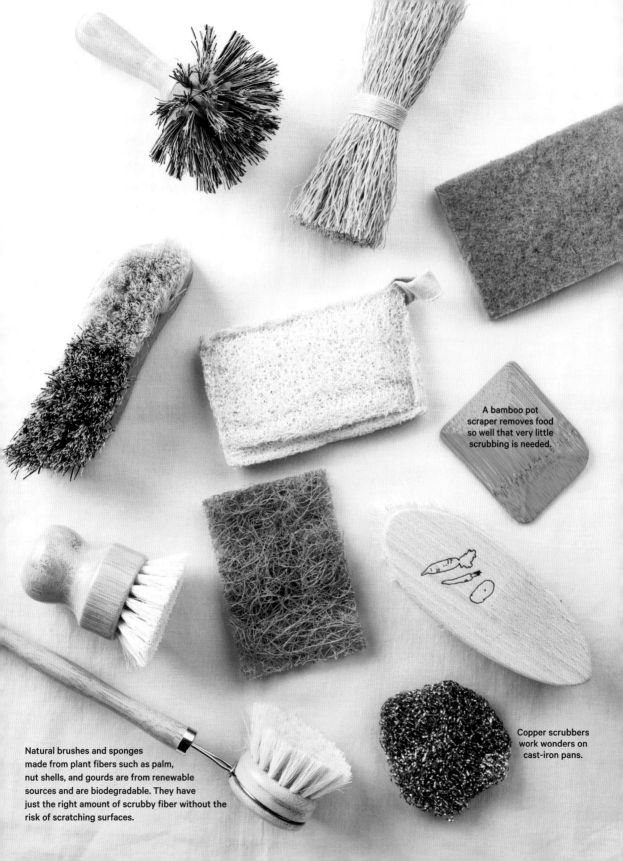

A bamboo pot scraper removes food so well that very little scrubbing is needed.

Copper scrubbers work wonders on cast-iron pans.

Natural brushes and sponges made from plant fibers such as palm, nut shells, and gourds are from renewable sources and are biodegradable. They have just the right amount of scrubby fiber without the risk of scratching surfaces.

DETOX CLEAN THE KITCHEN

A DETOXIFIED KITCHEN is an inviting one! While you are deep cleaning your kitchen, get into the nooks and crannies to remove dust, mildew, and moisture. Having each area of the kitchen sparkling clean is like a breath of fresh air.

Air

Open the windows to ventilate the kitchen. Our olfactory systems evolved to help us sniff out danger, so we have a keen sense of smell. When we smell something that we find offensive, it's usually because the source of the smell is not good for us. Odor is often our first clue to rotten food, a dead mouse, or a water-damaged area with mold. Follow your nose to the source and remove it. Then clean the area with Tea Tree Wash (page 21) to kill bacteria. Dry all areas well and use an air purifier if needed.

Oven

It's not important to clean the inside of an oven so that it looks brand new. Television commercials for caustic spray-on cleaners may give us this idea, but the goal in cleaning an oven is simply to remove any burnt material that may have dripped onto the elements or buildup that will continue to burn when the oven is on, creating smoke and PAHs. This can be done with Tub Scrub (page 21). It has just the right amount of abrasive and bubbles to clean an oven sufficiently.

To start, make sure your oven is off and cool. Lay down a drop cloth or newspaper on the kitchen floor. Remove the racks and place them on the drop cloth or newspaper. Use a short-bristled scrub brush and several tablespoons of Tub Scrub to scrub away the grime on the racks. Flip them over to scrub both sides. Use a wet rag to wipe off each side and repeat if necessary. To clean the interior of the oven, use a moist rag to apply Tub Scrub. Then rinse the interior surface by wiping it down with clean damp rags.

Ceiling, Walls, and Floor

Start high and work down. Remove light fixtures, clean out bugs and dust, and clean the glass. Dust, using a pole duster if needed to reach the ceiling. Kitchen walls build up a surprising amount of gunk from cooking oils, dust, and food splatters. If the walls are painted (rather than papered), spray them with Tea Tree Wash and wipe down with a clean dry cloth, replacing the cloth often to avoid spreading dust.

Finally, vacuum or sweep the floors, then wash the floor with Tub Scrub. Use a scrub brush or fibrous sponge if the floor has a buildup of residue. Use a mop if you have a large floor area. Then rinse the floor with a mop or clean damp cloths and dry well.

Cabinets and Countertops

Remove all items from each cabinet. Spray all surfaces with Tea Tree Wash, and dry well with clean rags. Be sure to get the tops of the cabinets, too, if they're accessible. Clean inside all drawers, all countertop surfaces, and the cabinet underneath the sink.

Cutting Boards

Sanitize all your cutting boards, as described on page 29. Use Tub Scrub for abrasive power, if needed. If your wooden cutting boards are damaged or rough, sand them smooth and apply a thin layer of vegetable oil to condition them.

Refrigerator

Remove everything from your fridge, washing any sticky condiment bottles with warm water and a clean towel. Wipe down all the shelves and drawers with Tea Tree Wash. Wipe down the exterior of the fridge, too, including the top if it's accessible. It's a good idea to make this a weekly habit, and it's a great time to organize and make a grocery list for the upcoming week.

Garbage Disposal

Mist Tea Tree Wash over all the surfaces of the disposal that you can access, then pour a kettle of boiling water down the drain. Run the disposal, with the cold water running, for 10 seconds to clean any material in the grinder mechanism.

Sink

Tub Scrub is the perfect cleaner and disinfectant for the sink. Use it at the end of the day to clean and polish the interior, faucet, and backsplash. Scrub, rinse, and dry with rags. Toss the used rags in a laundry basket.

Microwave

Spray the interior of the microwave with Tea Tree Wash and wipe down every surface, including those that are hard to see. Some microwaves have removable interior parts; be sure to wash them in the sink, and then dry and replace.

Pans

If degreaser is needed, use Sal Suds and hot water. If abrasion is needed, use Tub Scrub and a stiff fiber sponge or brush.

CERAMIC PANS. Nontoxic ceramic pans will remain nonstick as long as they don't have scratches or burned surfaces. However, if food does start to stick to one, you may need a little gentle abrasion. Add a few tablespoons of salt to the pan and use a soft cloth or sponge to scour away stuck food; the salt won't damage the nonstick surface of your pan.

CAST-IRON SKILLETS. Most cast-iron skillets are now pre-seasoned when you purchase them. Over time, that nice protective oily coating gets rinsed away and your pan will need to be reseasoned. This is important because cast iron will rust without a proper seasoning.

First, scrub the skillet in hot soapy water to remove gunk and any rust. Dry thoroughly.

Pour a tablespoon or two of olive oil on a small clean rag and wipe oil over all the surfaces of the pan. Wipe away any excess oil with a dry rag. Place a baking sheet on the lower rack of your oven and set the second rack in the middle of the oven. Preheat the oven to 375°F (190°C). Place the skillet upside down on the middle rack. Bake for 1 hour, then turn off the heat and let the pan cool in the oven.

After seasoning the skillet, avoid using soap when cleaning it to preserve the patina. Instead, scrub the cast iron with a brush or coarse salt, rinse, and dry well. That's it.

Trash Bin

Choose a trash bin that can be cleaned easily. Empty the bin, then spray it with Tea Tree Wash and wipe dry with a clean cloth. Use biodegradable bags and be sure to clean the inside of the can at least once a month to avoid mold growth.

CONGRATULATIONS!

You've detox cleaned the most complex room in the house. Light weekly cleanings will be enough to maintain this deeply cleaned room. Take a few deep breaths. What a difference! Enjoy preparing healthy meals in your fresh nontoxic kitchen.

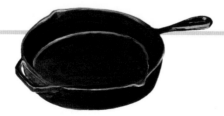

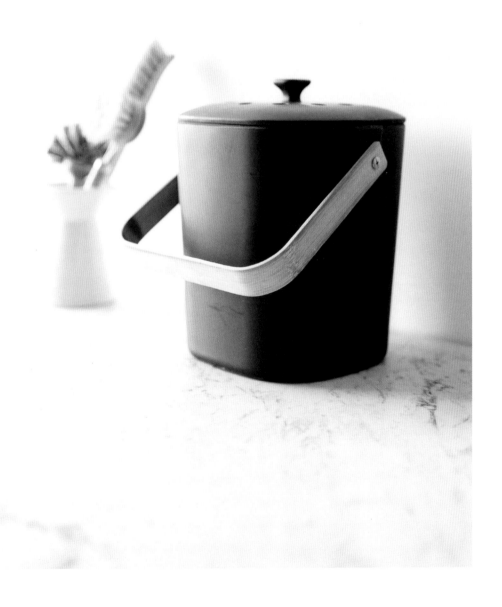

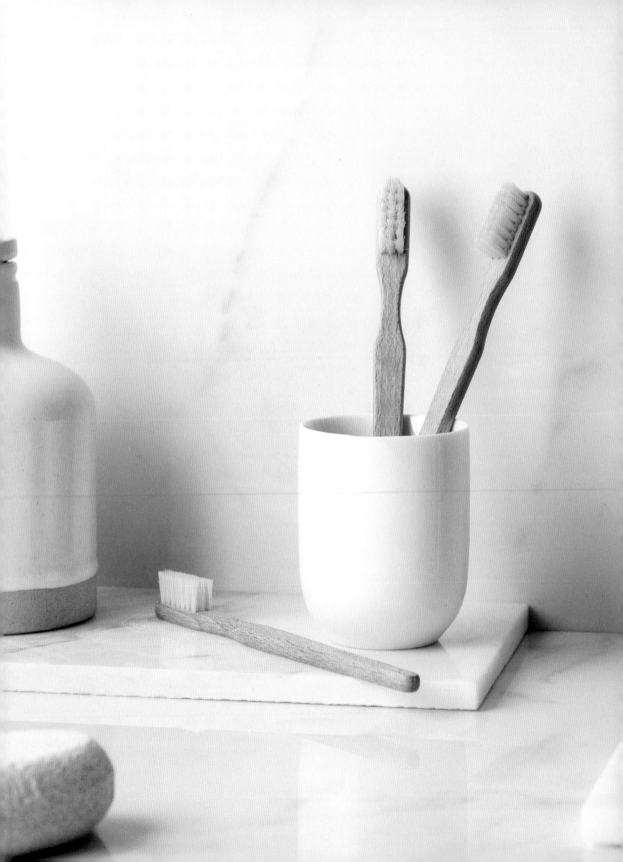

3
BATHROOM

A detox makeover of the bathroom can be tremendously beneficial to your family's health, simply because there are so many risks in this room. Many bathroom products are sources of potentially toxic chemicals, and the warm, humid environment of the bathroom is the ideal breeding ground for bacteria and mold.

HIDDEN TOXINS IN THE BATHROOM

YOUR DAILY SHOWER could mean a significant encounter with highly volatile toxins thanks to plastic shower curtains, memory-foam bathmats, mass-market hair products, and microorganisms that grow in your showerhead and on bathroom surfaces. As you work your way through the Toxic Ten, I'll draw your attention to some of the most toxic products, from cleaning sprays to accessories. As in the kitchen, read product labels carefully and look up any ingredients you don't recognize.

Give this space a thorough going-over and remove and replace everything that poses a risk to your health. We must cast a stern eye on every item, even those that seem comforting, like a cushy bathmat, soft towels, or a fancy showerhead.

Air Fresheners

Fresheners and deodorizers are among the worst indoor air pollutants we bring into our homes. Whether they are sprayed from a bottle, emitted from a plug-in, sprinkled onto a carpet, or burned as candles and incense, they release chemicals in a vaporized form that we then inhale through our lungs, ingest through our mouth, and absorb through our skin. These products are surprisingly harsh considering their common domestic use. They emit formaldehyde, phthalates, and volatile organic compounds (VOCs), and they trigger sensory irritation, respiratory symptoms, dysfunction of the lungs, damage to the central nervous system, cardiovascular and autoimmune issues, and hormone changes.

More than 20 percent of the population has severe and specific reactions to air fresheners and deodorizers. We may not think about these scented products as dangerous, but these "secondhand scents" raise concerns parallel to secondhand smoke. Short-term exposure to fragranced home products has been found to cause skin reactions, migraines, fatigue, respiratory irritation, visual disorders, asthma attacks, dizziness, nausea, allergic reactions, and loss of coordination. Long-term exposure has been proven to be carcinogenic and cause damage to the kidneys and liver, as well as the respiratory, endocrine, and central nervous systems.

An estimated 55 million adults in the United States have chemical sensitivity or multiple chemical sensitivity (MCS). Dr. Anne Steinemann at the University of Melbourne says, "MCS is a serious and potentially disabling disease that is widespread and increasing in the US population." Millions more suffer from conditions such as migraine headaches and asthma attacks that are triggered by exposure to fragranced products. More than 10 million people are considered disabled from these exposures. On top of that, millions lose workdays due to health problems from exposure to air fresheners and deodorizers. Clearly, the practice of using synthetic fragrances needs to be curtailed in our homes as well as public places.

Some of the VOCs released by air fresheners into the indoor environment, including xylene, aldehydes, benzene, and esters, are known to cause sensory irritation, migraine and tension headaches, respiratory symptoms, and dysfunction of the lungs.

TOXIC TEN

1. **AIR FRESHENERS**
2. **BACTERIA**
3. **BATH BOMBS**
4. **COSMETICS AND SKIN CARE**
5. **MENSTRUAL CARE**
6. **MOLD**
7. **ORAL CARE**
8. **PERFUMES**
9. **PLASTICS**
10. **TRICLOSAN**

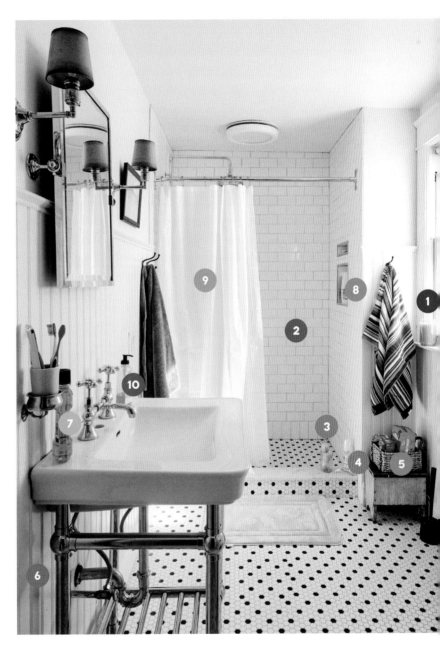

In addition, excessive exposure to benzene has been known for more than a century to damage bone marrow, resulting in a decrease in the numbers of circulating blood cells, and potentially aplastic anemia as well as leukemia.

When air fresheners emit these chemicals, they react with ozone to produce secondary pollutants such as formaldehyde, secondary organic aerosols (SOA), and ultrafine particles. These pollutants can cause damage to the central nervous system and act as endocrine-disrupting chemicals, altering hormone levels. On top of this, the ultrafine particles created by air fresheners can cause severe adverse effects to the lungs and cardiovascular systems. The more scented products in your home, the higher the risk. Studies have found that the deleterious health effects of air freshener chemicals may not manifest for many years, making it difficult to link these products to symptoms and disease.

Air fresheners are supertoxins. So why do we use them? Cleaning with nontoxic solutions removes the true source of offending odors, rather than masking them with toxic air freshener products. To begin, ventilate well by opening windows, and use an air purifier with a filter to remove airborne particles. Try the Essential Oil Spritzer (page 18) with a fresh-smelling essential oil, such as bergamot, citrus, lavender, or ylang ylang, to add natural nontoxic fragrance to your home. Skip the incense, which contains VOCs, and consider adding houseplants that are effective at pulling toxins out of the air.

KIDS, PETS, AND AIR FRESHENERS

Many health conditions suffered by children and pets can be tracked back to fragranced products in the home. I saw the effects of these products when I made a house call to a family who were all experiencing neurological issues and a number of other concerning symptoms. The minute I walked in the door, I was hit with many different strong smells, including dog urine, perfume, carpet powder, scented laundry soap and dryer sheets, and air fresheners. The family was using scented products to cover up strong pet odors. I recommended that they discontinue use of all deodorizers, air fresheners, and fragranced cleaning products, and hire a professional green cleaning service to tackle the walls and carpet, which they did. One of the children in the home had been suffering from mental health issues and reported feeling calmer and more focused after this deep cleaning. A teen in the house had been suffering from ADHD and hyperactivity. She reported a significant drop in her symptoms and, surprisingly, her nightmares vanished. The transformation in the health of their dogs was exciting. Both of their old dogs had more energy, and the carpet messes stopped completely.

Bacteria

Bathrooms are active rooms with water running, toilets flushing, showers misting, and people rushing in and out. We bring microbes into the room because there are trillions of them all over our bodies, and many of them end up on damp surfaces, where they start to replicate immediately. When we flush the toilet, tiny particles of poop and urine are misted into the air and settle on every surface, including towels, toothbrushes, and anything not tucked away in a drawer or cabinet. Not only bacteria but also viruses and fungi grow in fecal particles. So put your toothbrushes, towels, and cosmetics in cabinets, drawers, or closets if possible.

Makeup brushes pick up bacteria from our skin. So clean your brushes weekly with soap and a few drops of tea tree essential oil to kill bacteria, and if you have visible infections on your skin (acne), disinfect makeup brushes, dry brushes, face sponges, and towels after each use.

Bath Bombs

These invigorating multilayered explosions of color and scent release aldehydes, dyes, phthalates, parabens, and extremely toxic solvents, including benzene, into bathwater. Aldehydes have been linked to autism spectrum disorders and benzene to acute myeloid leukemia (AML), acute lymphocytic leukemia (ALL), chronic lymphocytic leukemia (CLL), multiple myeloma, and non-Hodgkin's lymphoma. I consider bath bombs supertoxins, right up there with air fresheners on the level of seriousness! Instead of using them, create luxurious and relaxing bath fragrance with a few drops of essential oil. Add Epsom salts for relaxation; we absorb magnesium from them as we soak, which reduces anxiety and tension.

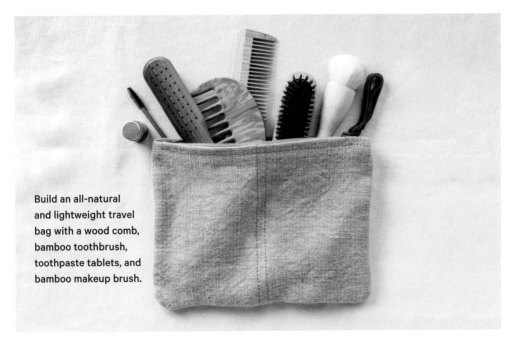

Build an all-natural and lightweight travel bag with a wood comb, bamboo toothbrush, toothpaste tablets, and bamboo makeup brush.

Cosmetics and Skin Care

We apply cosmetics and skin care products to some of the most sensitive and permeable parts of our bodies, so they have a direct effect on our health. The average woman puts 515 synthetic chemicals on her body every single day!

Various types of cosmetic products are so well studied now that we know exactly which ingredients cause cancer, heart disease, and diabetes. For example, parabens, which are in 20 percent of all personal care products, play a significant role in the development of gestational diabetes and have also been linked to immune diseases like allergies, asthma, and lupus. Products containing hydroquinone are used daily by 94 percent of all women and 69 percent of all men. Hydroquinone is a skin-bleaching agent that can damage skin, affect organs, and cause permanent corneal damage.

Fortunately, there are clean alternatives made from plant-based materials and minerals. Replace toxic cosmetic and skin care products with natural ones. Check the Environmental Working Group's cosmetic database, Skin Deep, for help in finding nontoxic products (see Resources, page 164).

If you ever suspect that you have negative symptoms, like asthma or migraines, connected to a personal care product, consider a total elimination test: Avoid the product completely for two weeks, then add it back to your routine and see what happens. With an elimination test, you assess one product at a time; this makes it easier to detect which products might be triggering symptoms.

EYE MAKEUP. The skin around our eyes is very delicate, and it absorbs any makeup we apply readily. Once the chemicals are in our bloodstream, the immune system sees them as foreign matter and responds by sending out white blood cells to engulf and destroy them. As those white blood cells attack, they bring fluid with them, and blood vessels become enlarged and red.

This whole process is our wondrous immune defense system working to clean up as much of these toxic chemicals as possible, but problems develop when inflammation gets out of hand. And this excess inflammation is at the root of most disease, so these little irritations, and even small daily exposures, can lead to damage in the body.

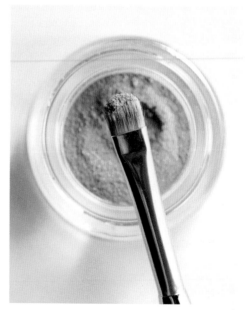

Mineral-based makeup products are generally free of toxic ingredients.

Since we don't have laws in place to keep companies from using health-damaging compounds, the burden lies with us to read labels. Eyeshadow, eyebrow pencil, and eyeliners often contain formaldehyde, microplastics (from glitter), parabens, talc, and even lead and coal tar. If you use eyebrow gel, also watch for aluminum. A friend, who is a professional model, told me something surprising: Top models avoid wearing eye makeup except when they're on a job. Wearing makeup daily often leads to eye inflammation, and that could keep models from being able to work, so they go makeup-free on their days off to protect their skin. This is great advice for us all. Skip the eye makeup except for special occasions.

Mascara is one of the most toxic cosmetics, with aluminum powder, coal tar dyes, formaldehyde, lead, mercury, parabens, synthetic dyes, and thimerosal (mercury-based preservative). Mascara also sheds particles that can irritate eye tissue and the corneas and cause sties and cysts. Mineral-based mascara is a nontoxic alternative. Look for mascara packaged in glass rather than plastic, and with clean ingredients like activated charcoal, aloe vera, bentonite clay, and vitamin E.

POWDERS. Talcum powder is a product that's been in use for decades, even on babies. It turns out this seemingly innocent stuff can cause ovarian cancer, testicular cancer, and mesothelioma. Magnesium silicate, the primary component of talc, can be carcinogenic when breathed in or absorbed through skin. Safer food-grade powders, like cornstarch and bentonite clay, can do the same job of absorbing sweat without the risky side effects.

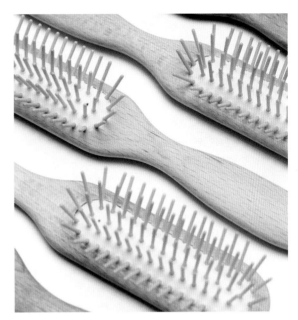

A wood hairbrush is more sustainable than plastic and won't rip your hair.

When researchers tested various facial powder products, from high-end brands down to the drugstore generics, they found parabens and talc in most of them. Mineral-based powders are our best option, as they are generally free of these toxic compounds.

HAIR TOOLS. Hair tools, including hair dryers, curling irons, flat irons, brushes, combs, and hair ties, are huge contributors to landfills due to their short lives and ever-changing styles that drive sales. Once in landfills, they degrade and release micro- and nanoplastics into the soil and atmosphere and become part of our planet's water cycle. They take hundreds of years to break down. Skip the daily drying and curling (except for special occasions) and look for eco-friendly alternatives made of biodegradable materials, like natural rubber hair ties and natural-bristle brushes with wooden handles, online and in natural foods stores.

HAIR SPRAY. If you need a little hair control now and then, try sea salt hair-spray products or organic sugar hair fixers.

SHAMPOO. Our skin is highly absorbent. When we apply lotions, soaps, and other personal care products, their ingredients are drawn right through our skin and into our bloodstream. That includes the skin on our scalp and the shampoos, conditioners, and other hair care products we use.

Shampoos contain a long list of ingredients, many of which are not good for us. Most have synthetic fragrances, dioxane, and phthalates. Some contain the neurotoxic diethanolamine. Many contain parabens, which are easily absorbed through the skin in those few minutes while we're washing our hair. Parabens are endocrine disrupters that affect hormones, fertility, and thyroid function. Studies have shown that when we use paraben products on our skin, they show up in breast milk and urine, proving that significant absorption is happening right through the skin. Parabens as well as fragrances can trigger asthma, even from short-term exposure through lungs and skin. So hair products, even those that we rinse out, matter to our health.

One solution is to buy more natural shampoo. You can often find good-quality, all-natural, liquid shampoo sold in bulk at co-ops and natural foods stores. Bring your own bottle to fill up and reuse. Solid shampoo bars are also a great option, and they usually come in paper packaging, not plastic. More than 600 million shampoo bottles end up in landfills every year. If we all stopped using them, we could save the planet from a mountain of plastic.

CONDITIONER. Conditioners often contain synthetic fragrances, parabens, and phthalates. Look for hair conditioner bars to avoid the plastic packaging. Or buy conditioner in bulk from your local food co-op; bring your own bottle and refill as needed.

LIPSTICK AND BALM. When I lived in Sun Valley, Idaho, I used lip products daily to protect my lips from sun exposure. When I looked into the ingredients, I was surprised to find that many of the products contained carcinogens. That's when I developed a passionate interest in learning about the ingredients used in consumer products. Lip balms often have a vast array of endocrine-disrupting chemicals, including parabens. Lipstick is even

---

WHAT DOES "NATURAL" MEAN?

I use the term natural *to describe products* that contain no synthetic chemicals and those made from natural materials such as minerals and plants. However, be aware that when manufacturers use the word *natural* on labels, it means nothing. There aren't any standards defining the use of the term on product packaging or in marketing. This means that a company can label any product *natural*. So beware. Read labels, do your research, and don't believe everything the companies tell you.

riskier; many commercial brands contain cadmium, lead, parabens, and phthalates.

As alternatives to the usual solid-color lipsticks, try beeswax-based versions with plant-based tints; they are generally cleaner. Look for lip balms made with edible ingredients in nonplastic packaging, such as paper tubes.

NAIL POLISH. Nail polish contains formaldehyde, toluene, and dibutyl phthalate (DBP), making it a risky habit. These chemicals damage the nervous system, increase plaque in arteries, and affect cognitive function, causing foggy brain. In 2012 the California Environmental Protection Agency evaluated 25 nail products, including nail polish, and found that 83 percent of the products that claimed to be toluene-free contained toluene at concentrations ranging up to 190,000 ppm (parts per million), and 14 percent of the products that claimed to be DBP-free contained DBP at concentrations ranging up to 88,000 ppm. Consider skipping nail polish altogether. If you want your nails to shine, use a natural buffer to give them a gleam.

NAIL POLISH REMOVER. Common ingredients in nail polish removers include acetone, ketones, propylene glycol, and synthetic fragrances and dyes, among many other toxins, and they may cause reproductive harm, neurological disorders, and organ toxicity—more reasons to skip the nail polish altogether.

DEODORANT AND ANTIPERSPIRANT. Deodorant and antiperspirant products contain a long list of toxins that are absorbed into the skin. The most common and concerning include aluminum, diethanolamine, parabens, phthalates, propylene glycol, triclosan, and triethanolamine. Look instead for deodorants with plant-based or natural ingredients such as baking soda and charcoal, which sorb to microbes. I search for those with sustainable packaging.

• ● •

TEA TREE DEODORANT

This simple deodorant wicks moisture and keeps you smelling clean all day long. Tea tree works to kill bacteria. Shea butter is the plant fat from the nuts of the shea tree. It's solid at room temperature and has an ivory color and an earthy scent.

5 tablespoons shea butter
5 tablespoons baking soda
½ teaspoon tea tree essential oil

Melt the shea butter in a small saucepan over medium heat. Remove from the heat and add the baking soda and essential oil. Mix well with a spoon and let the mixture cool until it is room temperature. Stir one more time and then scoop the mixture into a small jar with a lid. Use your fingers to apply a pea-size dollop to each armpit daily.

EXFOLIANTS. Many exfoliants contain microplastics, which have become a significant source of pollution in our waterways. Instead, try natural-fiber scrub sponges, cloths, or dry brushes, which gently exfoliate skin by removing dead skin cells.

The best exfoliation method for the planet and your skin is dry brushing, a technique developed over thousands of years through the Ayurvedic system in India. Use a natural-fiber brush to brush your dry skin in circular motions along lymphatic lines, which improves lymphatic drainage, circulation, and cellular detoxification. It is the most natural and effective way to remove dead skin cells, and it allows clogged pores to open up, releasing sebaceous oils that soften the skin and leave it glowing. Look for plastic-free dry brushes with plant-based fibers—soft bristles for your face and stiffer bristles for your body.

FACE WASH. Face wash products, like body soaps, contain damaging ingredients, including alcohol, parabens, and triclosan. Our skin holds a multitude of beneficial bacteria, and we need them to keep our skin looking and feeling good. Triclosan kills these healthy and symbiotic organisms and starts a cycle of poor skin health. Avoid it. Instead of facial wash, use a splash of cold water or a warm towel press when needed, and nothing more. French women have been practicing this for generations. I love the brilliant simplicity.

LOTION. Lotions are rife with synthetic chemicals, including diethanolamine, hydantoins, parabens, phthalates, synthetic fragrances, triclosan, and triethanolamine. One

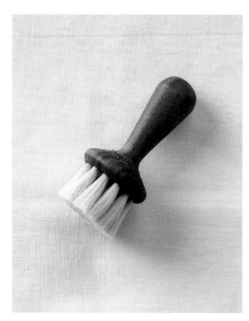

Dry brushing can improve skin health by removing dead cells and increasing circulation.

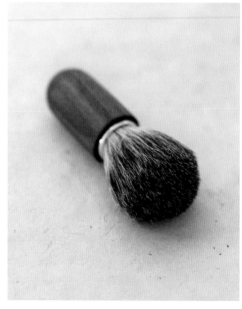

Well-made makeup and shaving brushes are beautiful and last for many years.

way to assess the ingredients in your skin care products is to think of your skin "eating" the products you put on it, and to act accordingly. In other words, do not apply anything to your skin that you would not eat or drink.

You may not need lotion at all, in fact. Dry brushing nightly stimulates the production of natural oils, which is often the only skin care habit you really need to keep your skin soft and smooth. If you have areas of severely dry skin and dry brushing isn't enough, apply a small amount of pure plant oil, such as shea, jojoba, or coconut oil. If you buy lotions, look for paraben-free products that contain only recognizable ingredients, like coconut oil, jojoba oil, and vitamin E.

RAZORS. The EPA estimates that two billion plastic razors are thrown away each year. In contrast, stainless-steel razors with replacement blades will last a lifetime. Even better is a Japanese straight blade, which can be sharpened and never needs a replacement blade.

SHAVING CREAM. Shaving creams and foams contain parabens, polyfluoroalkyl substances (PFAS), and triclosan, and their propellant is often ethanolamine, which has been shown to cause swelling in the brain. These toxic products are completely unnecessary. Natural bar soap works well for smooth shaving.

AFTERSHAVE. Aftershave products can contain hormone-disrupting chemicals including phthalates and VOCs. Ditch them in favor of pure aloe gel, which calms skin irritation and reduces inflammation.

SUNSCREEN. Many sunscreens contain chemicals that are toxic not only to us but also to our environment. Millions of people

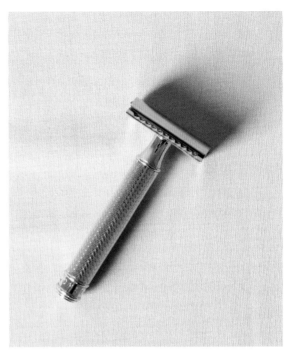

Using a metal razor helps decrease waste; the average person will throw away about 800 plastic razors in a lifetime!

wear sunscreen in the ocean every year, dispersing chemicals into the water. One of those chemicals is oxybenzone, a synthetic molecule known to be toxic to coral, algae, sea urchins, fish, and mammals. A single drop of this compound in four million gallons of water is enough to endanger ocean organisms. The great eco-warrior and Hawaii state senator Mike Gabbard authored legislation in 2018 to protect Hawaii's marine ecosystems by banning the dangerous sunscreen chemicals oxybenzone and octinoxate. This first-in-the-world law went into effect in January 2021.

In addition to oxybenzone and octinoxate, sunscreens often contain alkylphenols, ethanolamine, glycol ethers, parabens, phthalates, and triclosan. They have complex mixtures of endocrine-disrupting chemicals and asthma-related synthetic fragrances. These toxin-filled sunscreens are unnecessary because mineral-based products are safe and readily available and work well. Look for micronized zinc oxide and titanium dioxide, which create little umbrellas of impenetrable minerals that protect the skin, and products packaged in glass or cardboard tubes. And when it comes down to it, a hat is the best protection for your face—it blocks all UV rays.

MAKEUP REMOVER. If your makeup is natural, it will be water soluble, so you can use a warm, wet washcloth to remove it. Or you can use 100 percent organic cotton round pads with natural soap; they work well for removing makeup and can be washed and reused many times. Avoid the standard drug-store cotton balls. They are toxic little things that test positive for chlorine bleach, dioxins, plastics, polyester, polypropylene, and rayon. They are bad for our bodies and the environment. If you use ear swabs for wiping off makeup, be sure they are organic cotton, with a cardboard handle rather than plastic.

Menstrual Care

About 43 million people in the United States use tampons or pads. If you use them monthly, you will buy more than 11,000 in a lifetime. There should be ample information about the contents of these intimate products. However, as is the case for cosmetics, manufacturers of menstrual care products aren't required to tell us what's in them.

Toxins found in major brands include dioxins (carcinogenic), carbon disulfide (reproductive toxicant), hexane (neurotoxin), methylene chloride (carcinogen), toluene (reproductive toxicant), phthalates (endocrine disruptor), and xylene (neurotoxin, reproductive toxicant). Dioxins are a group of highly toxic chemical compounds that are associated with damage to the reproductive and immune systems. Dioxins are also damaging to the environment and known as persistent environmental pollutants (POPs) as they can remain in the environment for many years.

These products come in contact with some of the most sensitive and absorbent tissue in the body. They also frequently test positive for pesticides and bleach. All nonorganic products should be eliminated from use. Today, there are several alternatives for menstrual care, including washable and reusable pads, liners, and superabsorbent underwear, plus 100 percent organic cotton, nonchlorine, rayon-free, fragrance-free, and plastic-free products, and the reusable nontoxic silicone cup.

Mold and Mildew

Molds and mildews are types of fungi, and they're common in the warm, moist environment of bathrooms. Mold and mildew removal products are notorious for their long and varied list of noxious chemicals. But before we even look at the ingredients, our first clue is the warnings on their labels: *Do not inhale. Causes eye irritation. Do not get on skin or clothing.* Many labels outright tell consumers that the products are hazardous to humans.

The most environmentally sound, effective, and nontoxic way to remove mold and mildew is with antifungal essential oils like tea tree

MILDEW VS. MOLD

Mildew is a surface fungus that often lives on shower walls, windowsills, and other places where moisture levels are high, and it can easily be identified as a patch of gray or white fungal growth. Mold can be black or green and may appear fuzzy or slimy. Mildew and some molds can generally be removed easily, but some molds are harder to get rid of because the spores can grow deep in porous material.

and Tub Scrub (page 21), which is abrasive and will help remove fungus growing on tiles, shower enclosures, and shower curtains. Vinegar can also kill many types of molds and mildew, but it is acidic and can damage some kinds of grout.

Some molds can cause respiratory issues and act as neurotoxins. If people or animals in your home tend to be sick a lot and you have mold in your home, consider getting a test kit to determine whether it's a toxic variety.

Oral Care

Oral care products deserve special attention because anything we put on or in our mouths is absorbed readily into the bloodstream. We also swallow some of the products we use, such as toothpaste and mouthwash.

FLUORIDE. Fluoride calcifies and hardens teeth, but it affects other areas of the body, too. Fluoride exposure can cause calcification of the pineal gland, a tiny organ nestled in the brain. The pineal gland accumulates significant amounts of calcium and fluoride, making it the most fluoride-saturated organ in the human body. Both the calcification and accumulation of fluoride may result in melatonin deficiency, which affects sleep and is a contributing factor

to breast cancer development. Calcification of the pineal gland also reduces the organ's ability to communicate properly with the endocrine system, which can lead to health issues with the thyroid and pancreas.

Fluoride treatment is often part of bleaching treatments, but it may not be worth the risk. Having your teeth cleaned by a hygienist will remove plaque and tartar and likely reduce discoloration. Once the hard work is done, maintain your freshly cleaned teeth by brushing with a toothpaste made from baking soda or bentonite clay. Avoiding foods that stain teeth, like coffee, tea, and wine, will help your teeth stay bright without bleaching.

Some dentists also use fluoride treatments as part of regular dental care. If that's the case with your dentist, you may want to switch to a dental clinic that uses fewer toxic materials.

MOUTHWASH. A rinse to freshen the mouth should be simple and clean, but a quick review of popular mouthwash brands reveals a long list of unhealthy ingredients, including ethanol, fluoride, parabens, polyethylene glycol, and synthetic dyes.

Mouthwash is like air freshener—it's used to cover up odors rather than address the underlying issues. Foul breath is mainly caused by bacterial imbalance. Brush your teeth (and your tongue!) well and floss to remove any stuck bits of food that are feeding bacteria in your mouth, and you should be fine without mouthwash.

Activated charcoal powder is another simple product sold for use as a tooth polish and mouth freshener. It's simply finely ground charcoal and applied with a toothbrush. Wet your toothbrush, dip it into the charcoal powder, and then brush your teeth, gums, and tongue. The charcoal particles attach to bacteria and fungi and turn all hidden microbes black. Any bacteria caught in plaque along the gum line can be seen easily as black areas against white teeth, which helps guide your brushing to areas of bacterial growth that might otherwise be missed. Charcoal also absorbs live and dead microbes like a sponge so they can be rinsed out, which helps freshen the mouth.

If these tips don't do the trick, a visit to a nutritionist can provide guidance for improving diet and digestion. Probiotics for the gums and teeth can also help reduce pathogenic bacteria in the mouth, freshen breath, reduce inflammation in the gums, and reduce gum recession.

DENTAL FLOSS. Dental floss seems harmless, but many brands have the same toxic stuff that is used in Teflon: polytetrafluoroethylene (PTFE) and perfluorooctanoic acid (PFOA). These compounds are used to help floss slip easily between teeth. Floss is also often coated in plastics, which leave phthalate residue in your teeth. On top of that, floss often contains parabens and synthetic fragrances. Look for a natural brand made of cotton yarn or silk that is coated with plant-based wax, and packaged in glass or paperboard rather than plastic.

TOOTHBRUSHES. Toothbrushes should have soft bristles that are long enough to reach under the gums to remove food and bacteria. Up until recently we have accepted plastic toothbrushes as the norm. But they are

• ● •

MOUTH RINSE

An effective antibacterial mouth rinse can be made at home. Tea tree essential oil is antibacterial; peppermint also kills bacteria and tastes fresh and cool.

¼ cup water
2 drops tea tree essential oil
2 drops peppermint essential oil (optional)

Mix the ingredients and swish in your mouth for 20 seconds, which will kill many of the microbes that cause bad breath.

made from polyvinyl chloride (PVC), bisphenol A (BPA), numerous phthalates, polyethylene, and triclosan, so they are inherently toxic.

Since toothbrushes are disposable, they create a huge waste problem. Close to four billion brushes are sold worldwide each year, and a billion of them are thrown away in the United States annually, which equals 50 million pounds of plastic waste. To protect your health and the planet, make a switch to plastic-free, biodegradable bamboo toothbrushes with natural bristles.

TOOTHPASTE. Commercial toothpastes sold in plastic tubes have many questionable ingredients, including artificial sweeteners, diethanolamine, fluoride, microplastics, polyethylene, propylene glycol, and salicylate (aspirin). As an alternative, look for chewable toothpaste tablets and powders that come in glass or waxed paper bags or natural versions of toothpaste. Again, we can turn to tea tree essential oil, too, which inhibits pathogenic bacteria, making it an excellent addition to toothpaste. It is also an excellent disinfectant for toothbrushes.

WHITENING STRIPS. The European Union and Canada classify hydrogen peroxide, the whitening ingredient in commercial teeth

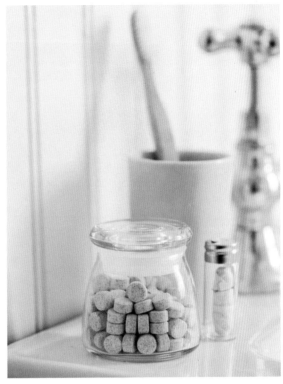

Toothpaste tablets, bamboo toothbrushes, and floss packaged in glass are plastic-free, nontoxic, low-waste choices for these everyday items.

whitening strips, as toxic or harmful when used in the mouth. It can destroy the oral microbiome, killing off the beneficial bacteria that prevent cavity formation, gum disease, bad breath, and other conditions.

GUM INFLAMMATION

Inflammation in the gums indicates infection, which means bacteria are present. One simple treatment is aloe vera gel, which can be harvested fresh from an aloe vera leaf. The gel can also be used as a salve for gum irritation and disease. It is nature's soothing healer, not only for sunburns but also for periodontal disease. Its anti-inflammatory properties reduce plaque-induced gingivitis.

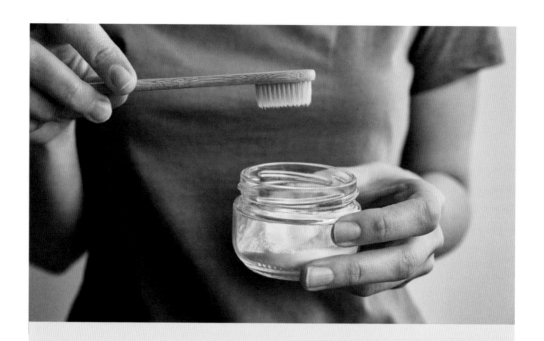

• • •

PEPPERMINT TOOTHPASTE

Baking soda removes stains, stevia balances the salty soda, tea tree kills bacteria and freshens breath, peppermint gives a bright flavor, and coconut oil is a smooth organic base. This recipe is intended for adults, as the essential oils may be too intense for children. A 6-year-old friend tried this toothpaste and exclaimed, "It's a bit too spicy for me!"

3 tablespoons coconut oil
3 tablespoons baking soda
1 teaspoon peppermint essential oil
1 teaspoon tea tree essential oil
10 drops liquid stevia

Melt the coconut oil in a small saucepan over medium heat. This takes only a minute or two. Remove from the heat and add the baking soda, peppermint essential oil, tea tree essential oil, and stevia. Mix well with a spoon and let the mixture cool until it's at room temperature. Stir one more time and then scoop the mixture into a small jar with a lid. You now have nontoxic toothpaste.

Sodium hydroxide is also common in whitening strips and considered a caustic agent, meaning it corrodes what it touches. It is also used in hair dye, and just like it strips the natural oils from hair, making it brittle, it strips the natural coating from teeth, making them more sensitive. PEG-8 is another component worth special mention, as it may cause hives upon contact with sensitive tissue like the cheeks, gums, or tongue. The Environmental Working Group warns that PEG-8 itself is also frequently contaminated with more dangerous chemicals like dioxane, a potential carcinogen.

The easiest natural method to whiten your teeth is to mix a tablespoon of baking soda with a tablespoon of water in a small bowl. Brush all surfaces of your teeth with this paste about twice a month. If you prefer commercial teeth-whitening products, look for those based on activated charcoal or baking soda.

Perfumes

Concentrated fragrances, perfumes, and cologne carry parabens, phthalate esters, solvents, and VOCs. These products, even the expensive ones, can easily pass through the skin and into the body, where their chemical components can affect the endocrine system. In some people, synthetically fragranced products can trigger migraine attacks after a few minutes of exposure. You can reduce your risk of negative effects by using perfume only on occasion and spraying it on your clothes rather than directly on your skin. As a non-toxic alternative, some essential oils are made as ready-to-use fragrances or you can blend

them yourself; be sure to dilute them with water and research which oils are safe to use.

Plastics

We use an enormous number of packaged products that create waste in the bathroom—all the tubes and bottles for deodorant, shampoo, cosmetics, and so on. More than 120 billion units of packaging are produced every year by the cosmetics industry. Recycling centers are maxed out, so many of these plastic containers go to landfills. But now many landfills are full, and a lot of the plastic ends up in the ocean, where it pollutes the water with micro- and nanoplastics and all their chemical components. Plastics are responsible for more than 80 percent of the negative effects on animals associated with ocean trash. The tiniest particles are now part of our atmosphere and found in every drop of rain. To stop this cycle, we must change our buying habits. A good starting place is the bathroom, the source of so much plastic waste. It is possible to set up a bathroom without any plastic at all by using things like a wood-handled toilet brush, shampoo bars, and paperboard lip balm tubes.

SHOWER CURTAINS. You know that heady plastic smell that fills the room after you unwrap a new plastic shower curtain? Well, what you are smelling are highly toxic chemicals including vinyl, phthalates, and other harmful substances. One study found that over the course of 28 days, a new plastic shower curtain releases 108 different VOCs. Over the course of its life, shower curtain vinyl emits toxins that cause inflammation and fatigue. If the curtain isn't cleaned regularly, mold grows along the bottom and in the folds and the mold breaks down the plastic faster, releasing more phthalates into the air.

If you have a plastic or vinyl shower curtain, consider replacing it as soon as possible. You could keep the old curtain in the garage to use as a tarp for messy projects. Replace it with a 100 percent organic cotton or linen shower curtain.

MEMORY-FOAM BATHMATS. Synthetic memory foam is a supertoxin! Rather than a memory foam bathmat, try a 100 percent organic cotton rug or bamboo bathmat, both of which can be tossed in the washing machine and washed with hot water and a few drops of tea tree essential oil to disinfect.

TOWELS. Many inexpensive towels are now made of synthetic materials that release phthalates and polyester into the environment. I recently bought a few nice-looking recycled towels, but when I used them, they caused a bumpy red rash all over my body. This was likely due to the mix of chemicals that end up in the plastic recycling process. Until the current contamination issue is resolved with recycled plastics, opt for organic cotton or linen towels.

Triclosan

Triclosan was initially developed as a surgical scrub for medical professionals, but it is now added to a slew of consumer products as an antimicrobial agent to kill bacteria and fungi and prevent odors. It may sound like a helpful ingredient, but the problem is that it kills not only pathogenic bacteria (the kind that cause disease) but also beneficial bacteria (the kind

we need to survive). In 2016 the FDA banned the use of triclosan in consumer soaps and body washes, noting that it is not generally recognized as safe or effective in these products.

Washing your hands or body with plain soap and water is as effective in removing bacteria as washing with a soap containing triclosan. But it is still an ingredient in some antibacterial soaps, hand sanitizers, and other products. We're ingesting triclosan from our toothpaste, toothbrushes, and tooth-whitening products and absorbing it through our skin from antiperspirants and deodorants, cosmetics, creams, lotions, and shaving products. It is also in a surprising number of household items, including detergents, spray cleaners, fabrics, kitchen cutting boards, shoes, toys, and other plastics.

This level of exposure is unsafe. In one study, the CDC identified triclosan in the urine of 75 percent of the people it tested. This level of exposure can cause a mass die-off of the microbes we need to help us digest food, support immune function, regulate mood, and perform hundreds of other critical biological activities that our bodies can't do properly without our essential microbes. When our beneficial microbe levels are reduced, we start to develop issues like poor digestion, susceptibility to infections, mood disorders, and hormonal imbalance. Overexposure to triclosan is now even linked to the development of diabetes because a reduction of essential microorganisms means improper digestion and metabolism, which puts a strain on the pancreas. The abundant use of triclosan is also leading to microbial antibiotic resistance.

Even in low concentrations, triclosan can trigger antibiotic resistance in bacteria and fungi.

Avoid triclosan in all your products, bathroom-related or not. Read labels carefully, as triclosan can also be called 2,4,4-trichloro-2-hydroxydiphenyl ether, trichloro-2-hydroxydiphenyl ether, 5-chloro-(2,4-dichlorophenoxy) phenol, CH-3565, or TCS.

TRICLOSAN AND PETS. Triclosan is used in pet products, too. When animals come in contact with household items that contain triclosan, they ingest and breathe these chemical molecules, which has been proven to be harmful to their health. In dogs, it kills the beneficial microbes in their noses, which causes inflammation, alters blood flow, interferes with their hydration, and reduces their sense of smell by interfering with their olfactory receptors. Because scents are behavioral stimuli for dogs, this can affect their behavior. Triclosan also affects animal digestion and increases pets' risk for pathogenic infections.

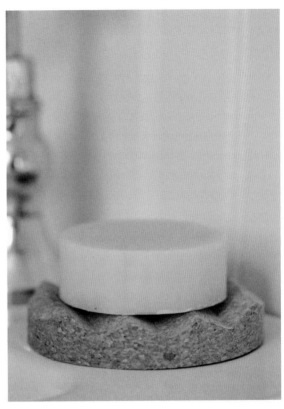

Replace plastic with sustainable materials such as a renewable cork soap dish.

ANTIVIRAL HAND SANITIZER

During a global pandemic viral outbreak, hand sanitation is vital. However, researchers found that washing hands thoroughly with hot water and soap is more effective than using hand sanitizer products with triclosan. For times when hand washing is not possible, diluted tea tree oil can be an effective antimicrobial agent.

DETOX CLEAN THE BATHROOM

NOW THAT YOU'VE UNCLUTTERED and removed all toxic items from your bathroom, you're ready to clean away any residual chemicals and microbes that are left behind. A quick reminder: Odors are generally from organic matter like poop, urine, and bacteria. The 400 million cans of toxic deodorizers and air fresheners that are sold each year only mask smells, rather than addressing the underlying issue. Only by removing the source of the offending odor can you truly eliminate bad bathroom smells.

To save time, energy, and environmental resources, I recommend taking a few minutes each evening to tidy up and wipe down counters, faucets, and other surfaces. Pick up dirty clothes and wet towels and place them in a laundry basket. Do a deep cleaning once a week, beginning with the walls, light fixtures, and shelves and working your way down to the lowest and grubbiest areas, including the tub, toilet, and floors.

Air

Make sure your bathroom has a ventilation fan and turn it on when you shower to help vent moisture and airborne toxins. If you have a window, open it for further ventilation. What if you don't have a vent or window? Place a small bowl of baking soda on a shelf or the back of the toilet, where it can absorb moisture and odors. Replace it weekly.

Bathtub

Use Tub Scrub to remove scum and disinfect all surfaces. Use a cloth, scrub sponges, or a brush to help remove soap buildup. Rinse well.

Bathmat

Assuming that your bathmat is washable (which it should be!), run it through the washing machine. Use a natural laundry soap and add a few drops of tea tree essential oil to kill fungi and odors, or make your own Liquid Laundry Soap (page 19).

Drains

Prevent clogs with a wire mesh, stainless-steel, or silicone drain catcher. If your drain is already blocked, avoid commercial drain cleaners, as they are highly reactive and full of caustic chemical dissolvers that damage pipes and are toxic to people, ocean animals, and the environment. A safer alternative is to thread a drain snake into the drain to remove hair, buildup, and other debris.

Medicine Cabinet

Pare down your medicine cabinet by eliminating all items that are past their expiration date and any products or medications you no longer use. If you're getting rid of medications, take them to your pharmacy for proper disposal rather than flushing or tossing them as they are a surprisingly significant source of pollution in our water supply.

Remove all items from the cabinet shelves and mist all surfaces with Tea Tree Wash, then dry thoroughly with a clean cloth. As you put everything back into the cabinet, consider how much you use each item and whether it is toxin-free. Replace any products that have questionable ingredients, like antiperspirant containing aluminum.

Shower

Use Tub Scrub to polish and disinfect the shower, including the shower door, if you have one, and its tracks. An old toothbrush is handy for tackling tough spots like tile grout and corners. A natural scrub brush is an excellent tool for making quick work of the entire shower enclosure. Be on the lookout for dark spots, as they're a sign of mold and mildew growth. To remove, coat the spot with a small amount of Tub Scrub and let it seep in, so it penetrates below the surface and reaches even the deepest mildew spores. Scrub off with a brush or sponge. Rinse thoroughly.

Showerhead

A showerhead is a vector for microbes and a daily contamination source. Rob Dunn's book *Never Home Alone* goes into detail about the fascinating organisms that share our homes with us, such as mycobacteria that grow readily in the biofilm inside our showerheads. To clean and remove the biofilm that inevitably builds up inside, remove the showerhead and soak it in vinegar to break down any limescale, then scrub with a brush and Tub Scrub. The tea tree essential oil in the scrub will help eliminate the biofilm and its microbes. If you can, add a charcoal filter to your existing showerhead, which will remove microbes from the water, and be sure to change the filter annually.

Shower Curtain

Launder cloth liners and curtains in hot water with liquid soap and 10 drops of tea tree essential oil, and wash on the gentle cycle at least twice a month to remove mildew and bacteria.

Sink

Use Tub Scrub and a clean cloth to polish and disinfect the sink, faucets, backsplash, and other surfaces.

Surfaces

Spritz all surfaces with Tea Tree Wash to disinfect, including walls, counters, floors, baseboards, shelves, cabinets, and the inside of all drawers, and dry them with a clean cloth. Viruses are transmitted through the biological spatter that comes mainly from toilets as well as bathroom sinks and showers. These little liquid droplets end up on every surface area in the bathroom, which is why it's so important to thoroughly clean all surfaces with Tea Tree Wash, an effective pathogen cleanser.

Tiles

Tub Scrub works wonders on tile and grout. Scrub tiles with Tub Scrub and a brush, then rinse. If you see any mold, spray Tea Tree Wash on the area, let it sit for about 10 minutes, and then scrub and rinse. White vinegar is effective for removing mold and mildew on glass tub enclosures and bathtubs, but it may be too acidic for use on grout, stone tile, slate, granite, quartz, natural marble, or cultured marble made from stone and resin.

Toilet

Use Tub Scrub to polish and disinfect the toilet bowl. Mist Tea Tree Wash on all the outside surfaces and the floor immediately around the toilet, then wipe them dry with rags. Brushes work best for cleaning areas with bolts and latches. After use, disinfect brushes by rinsing

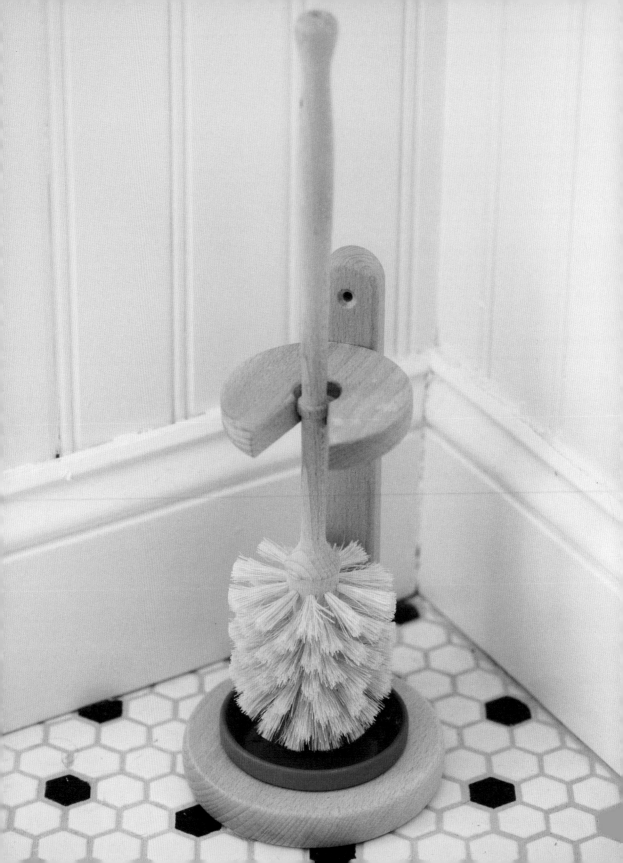

them in the tub, then misting the bristles with Tea Tree Wash. If you see lime or mineral deposits in the toilet, pour about 2 cups white vinegar into the toilet water and let it sit for an hour. This will help break down the mineral deposits to be scrubbed away.

TOILET PAPER. Trees are no longer a sustainable option for toilet paper material. And recycled toilet paper has its own issues as it contains BPA from contamination during the recycling process. It also may contain numerous phthalates, chlorine, parabens, phenols, inks, dyes, perfume, and triclocarban. Use 100 percent biodegradable toilet paper made completely from bamboo, a fast-growing, renewable, and nontoxic resource. The other option is a bidet; there are inexpensive add-on components for your toilet, which makes toilet paper unnecessary.

TOILET BOWL CLEANERS. Toilet bowl cleansers contain sodium hypochlorite, ammonia, petrochemical solvents, bromine, and corrosive ingredients that create caustic fumes and release environmentally damaging toxins into our waterways and oceans. They are some of the most damaging chemicals used in our homes. Common ingredients in toilet bowl cleaning products disrupt hormone levels, modify estrogen and androgen signaling, affect fetal brain development, and increase the risk of neurodevelopment disorders. By replacing this one product with natural cleaning methods, you are making a significant improvement in your home and protecting the environment.

· ● ·

TEA TREE ANTIBACTERIAL SPRITZER

Unpleasant bathroom smells are caused by bacteria. Tea tree essential oil is a natural antibacterial and air freshener; just give a spritz in the air as needed. You can add fragrance to the formula with an essential oil like eucalyptus, which has an invigorating scent.

¼ cup water
1 teaspoon tea tree essential oil
2 drops essential oil of your choice, for fragrance (optional)

Combine the ingredients in a spray bottle, shake, and spritz as needed.

Windows and Mirrors

Clean windows and mirrors with Glass Spray (page 18). If there's visible mildew on or around windows, remove it by spraying Tea Tree Wash and then wiping dry with a clean cloth. This removes the mildew and helps inhibit future growth.

Window Coverings

Any fabric in a moist environment will likely have some mildew on it. Window curtains can be laundered with shower curtains. If you have blinds or shutters, mist every surface with Tea Tree Wash and wipe down with dry cloths to remove all particles of dust, mildew, and toxins. Paper blinds can't be washed because they are too delicate and many fall apart in water. If you have dirty paper blinds, they may need to be replaced.

GOOD WORK!

Now that you have removed the sources of odors, disinfected all surfaces, and cleaned everything of spills and splatters, your bathroom is a truly clean and safe sanctuary. You can add a fresh scent with an Essential Oil Spritzer using your choice of essential oils, like lavender, bergamot, peppermint, or rose. Feel a sense of peace in knowing that the space you are in, the products you use, and the air you breathe are supporting your health and well-being.

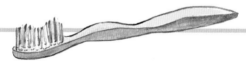

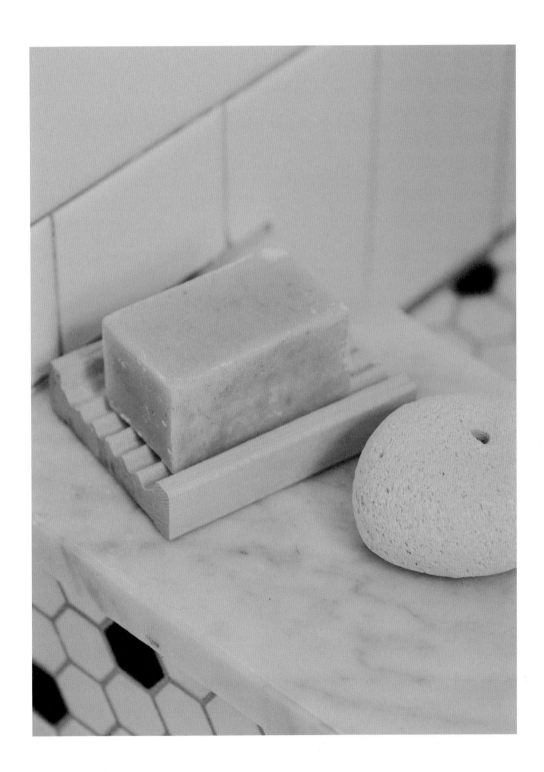

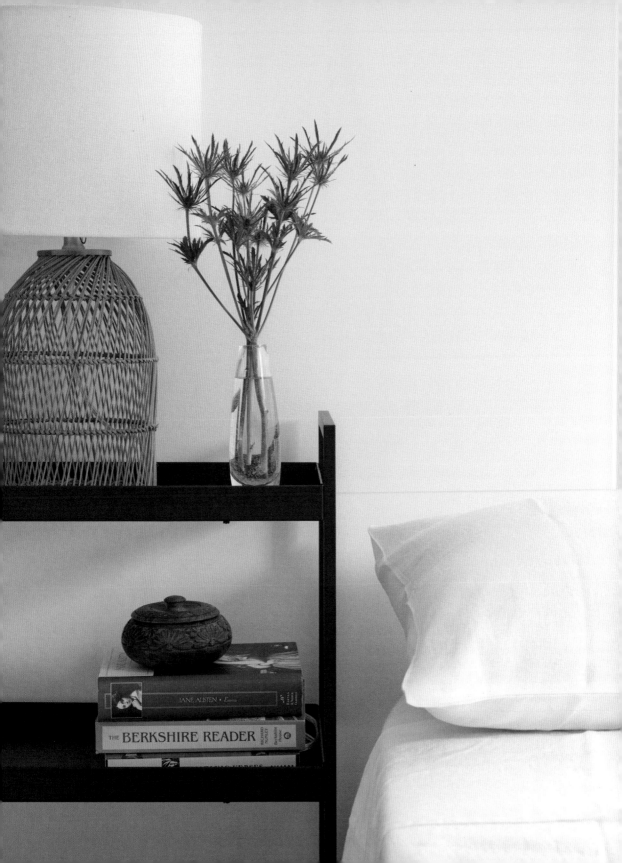

4

BEDROOM

Our bedrooms play a vital role in our overall health, due in part to the amount of time we spend in them. If we don't sleep well, we miss out on the restorative processes we need to be at our best. One way to make sure we sleep well is to keep the bedroom free of irritants, toxins, and other hidden sources of concern, including EMFs, mold, dust, and airborne chemicals.

HIDDEN TOXINS IN THE BEDROOM

OUR UNDERSTANDING of which materials are best for beds and bedding is changing quickly as we become more informed about the toxins in foam and other synthetics. Many beds bombard us with chemicals and unhealthy elements that contribute to disease, which makes it particularly important to thoroughly detoxify the bedroom.

Bedding

Sheets, blankets, duvets, and duvet covers are often made from a combination of cotton and synthetic materials. Read labels carefully before purchasing and look for organic and 100 percent cotton or linen. These natural fibers allow for changes in body temperature due to airflow through the woven threads, and they absorb moisture well.

To avoid synthetic materials like microfiber, which is plastic, keep an eye out for names that secretly tell you that an item is plastic; they often include the word "fil," like Pluma-fil.

Since sheets and textile materials require no government regulations, look for independent certifications like the ones listed below to help you know you're getting safe materials. Please note these organizations are not endorsing the text in this book; these are my personal recommendations.

 GLOBAL ORGANIC TEXTILE STANDARD (GOTS) is internationally recognized as having the toughest organic textile standards because it goes beyond verifying the organic farming process to include every

step of manufacturing. Products in the Organic category must contain 95 to 100 percent organic fiber, use nontoxic dyes, and not be treated with bleach, formaldehyde, or any other toxic substances; products in the Made with Organic category must reach at least 70 percent of those standards. Strict social and environmental standards are also required.

 STANDARD 100 BY OEKO-TEX® certifies that every component of a product has been tested for harmful substances and that the product is harmless for human health.

 MADE SAFE is an independent certification that ensures products are nontoxic by screening for a wide range of carcinogens, endocrine disruptors, heavy metals, and more.

 GREENGUARD GOLD certification helps assure that products designed for indoor spaces meet strict chemical emissions limits and take into consideration the reduced tolerance of sensitive individuals, including children and the elderly.

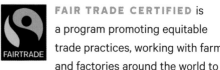 **FAIR TRADE CERTIFIED** is a program promoting equitable trade practices, working with farms and factories around the world to empower workers and improve wages, benefits, and conditions.

TOXIC TEN

1. BEDDING
2. BED FRAMES
3. CLOTHES
4. DUST
5. ELECTRONICS
6. MATTRESSES
7. MEMORY FOAM
8. MOLD
9. MOTHBALLS
10. PILLOWS

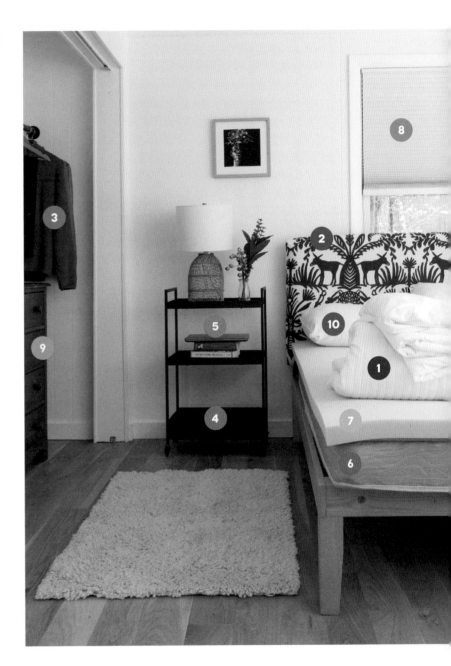

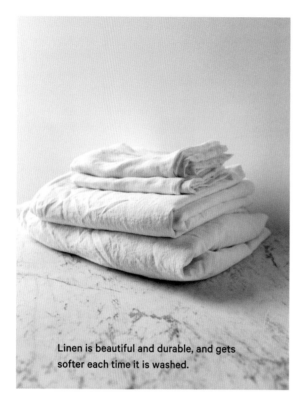

Linen is beautiful and durable, and gets softer each time it is washed.

Our beds are ideal environments for a vast menagerie, including mites, fleas, mold, bacteria, and fungi. Many of these organisms are asthma triggers and can exacerbate autoimmune and inflammatory conditions. If you are experiencing symptoms such as bites, itching, puffy eyes, and inflammation, clean your bedroom often. Once a week, wash your sheets, comforter, blankets, mattress pad, and pillows in a washing machine with hot water, soap, and an antimicrobial, such as 10 drops of tea tree, oregano, or thyme essential oil. Once a month, lift the mattress and box spring out of the frame, vacuum (with a HEPA filter) any dust from the frame and the floor, and wipe down the frame with Tea Tree Wash (page 21).

If air quality is an issue because you are particularly sensitive to it or because you live near a busy road or in a city, a HEPA air purifier can help.

PET BEDDING

Dog beds and cat cozies often contain brominated flame retardants, triclosan, arsenic, formaldehyde, phthalates, dioxins, and heavy metals and emit volatile organic compounds (VOCs). These chemicals can affect pets' neurological systems and have been found to cause epilepsy in dogs and hyperthyroidism in cats.

It's difficult to find bedding for animals that is natural and sustainable, so the safest solution is to create your own by wrapping a cotton blanket around some old pillows, stacking folded blankets, or folding an old down comforter into the right size for your pet. Natural nontoxic rubber dog mattresses are available, and they can offer much relief for older pets with stiff joints. Wash pet bedding with hot water, laundry soap, and a few drops of tea tree essential oil to help kill any fleas, ticks, bacteria, and mold.

Bed Frames

Many contemporary "wood" bed frames are made from composite materials, usually wood particles that have been fused together with plastics and glue. Composite and laminated woods have significant emission rates of VOCs, including toluene and terpenes. New bed frames off-gas at the highest level, but the rate of emission drops over time.

Padded headboards may look warm and inviting, but they are almost always made from foams and fabrics that are impregnated with flame retardants and formaldehyde. Sleeping with your face near these foams is a direct exposure to VOCs that cause oxidative stress and decrease lung function by triggering airway inflammation. Also, keep in mind that the fabric is difficult to clean, so it collects dust, dead cells, and all the same detritus as pillows over time.

If you're looking for a new bed frame, consider an unfinished solid wood frame and finish it yourself with a nontoxic sealer, vegetable dye, or stain. Metal frames are also a decent option as they are generally inert, although antiques could be coated with lead paint. Simple bed frames, such as platform beds, are easiest to clean because there is less surface area to vacuum and dust. And beds with replaceable parts can be repaired over time rather than being tossed out when a part wears out or gets damaged.

If you're buying a used bed frame, make certain that you are purchasing from a non-smoker, as any porous material like wood will have absorbed the smoke, cadmium, and VOCs along with it.

Clothing

Many clothing items are now treated with brominated flame retardants (BFRs) and also test high for heavy metals, formaldehyde, bisphenols, and phthalates. On top of that, many clothes are made of plastic. I walked through a store recently and looked at dozens of items. Some were soft like cashmere, some looked and felt like silk, and others mimicked wool, and they were all so affordable. When I checked the labels, though, I found more chemicals than I thought possible. The natural-looking fabrics were all made from synthetic materials, like polyamide, a plastic that has been found to contain high levels of lead. I looked at the store's clothing offerings online and saw they are made of acrylic, elastane, imitation leather (plastic), polyester, and petroleum-based viscose.

In textiles, formaldehyde is used to increase wrinkle resistance and to help dyes better penetrate. Formaldehyde—if you took a biology class you might remember that horrible smell—has been found to cause myeloid leukemia in those who work with the stuff. I ordered jeans from a popular clothing store, and when they arrived, they came with a warning (California Proposition 65) about formaldehyde's toxicity, and they really stunk, just like biology class. That experience spurred my investigation into a whole new arena of the toxins hanging in our closets. I learned that when we wear clothes that have been treated with formaldehyde, even many months after manufacturing, our warm, moist skin draws this chemical right into our bloodstream. The chemical legacy extends beyond the simple matter of our own exposure. When we wash this fabric, the formaldehyde leaches into our water system, where it then affects wildlife.

Thanks to California Proposition 65, products made with formaldehyde now carry a warning label stating: This product contains chemicals known to the State of California to cause cancer and birth defects or other reproductive harm.

THE TOXIC PRICE OF FAST FASHION

The volume of clothing purchased each year by Western consumers is about 400 percent more than it was a generation ago. The term "fast fashion" refers to clothes that are trendy for a season and then suddenly out of fashion. Some are then sent to thrift stores, but most end up in landfills, where BFRs, formaldehyde, heavy metals, solvents, and other toxins leach into the ground and into the water system.

When we buy toxic clothes, we breathe in the volatile gases emitted by the synthetic fabrics, and our skin absorbs toxic compounds from them at an alarmingly high rate. Blood tests show that we take these poisons into our bodies through our skin just as readily as if we had ingested them.

This affects not only consumers but also the people involved in manufacturing the clothing. All these toxins are being used in factories around the world where the outflow from production pours into water systems and the air, exposing local communities to these poisons.

One of the best ways to avoid this toxic fashion trap is to stop buying off the rack. If you need new clothes, shop at thrift or vintage clothing stores or organize clothing swaps with friends. Make your own clothing, and mend clothing that needs repair rather than tossing it. If you are buying new, buy higher quality rather than more items. When you find yourself needing a new item, take the time to research the option that is best for your health and the environment. Progressive clothing companies are creating eco-friendly and non-toxic items, and several shoe companies make durable yet biodegradable shoes.

ETHICAL, SUSTAINABLE, AND NONTOXIC FASHION

Nontoxic fabric options include organic cotton as well as bamboo, flax/linen, hemp, lyocell, silk, and wool. The greenest fabrics are those made from renewable fibers that require limited water and energy to produce. As with most things, quality makes a difference when you're buying new clothes. Look for well-made pieces with high-quality natural materials like silk, wool, and linen, and you'll be able to keep them for years.

BAMBOO. There are pros and cons to using bamboo as fiber. This fast-growing plant requires no pesticides to grow and produces machine-washable soft fabrics. However, turning its fibers into fabric requires some chemical processing.

COTTON. Most cotton fabric is nonorganic and grown with intensive use of agricultural chemicals. However, organic cotton is grown without the use of pesticides or herbicides. Also, organic cotton can be grown using 91 percent less water than its nonorganic counterpart when the crop is rain-fed rather than irrigated.

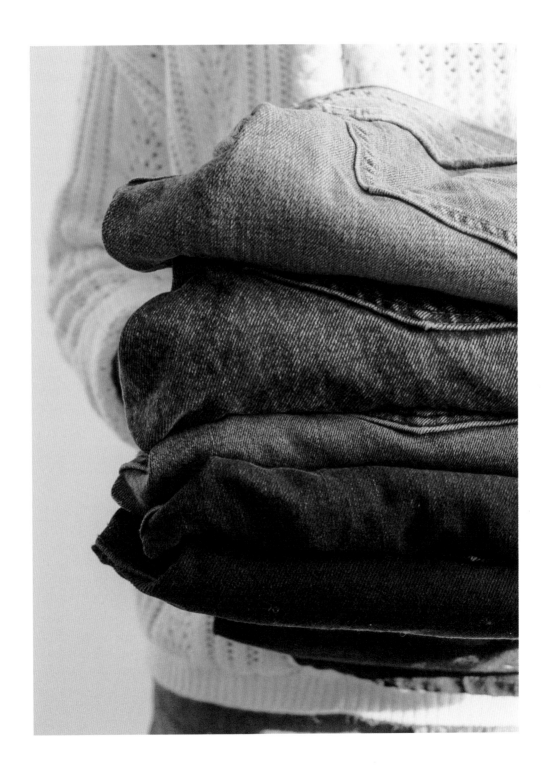

UPCYCLING AND REPAIRING

The "distressed" look in jeans means holes and rips. Distressed jeans are fashionable, but they get tossed in the garbage as soon as the holes get too big and the jeans start to fall apart. Repairing holes with visible mending is a way to give your clothing a new life. It's also meditative and enjoyable to relax into mending while watching a movie or sitting in the sun. The Japanese sashiko technique takes the idea of visible mending to an art form. Sashiko needles are like long embroidery needles, and the cotton sashiko thread has a more natural, rougher, grippy texture. The stitches settle into the fabric as solid little lines about the size of a grain of rice, and the end result is a gorgeous form of embroidery—and a mended piece of clothing that is wearable again.

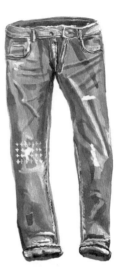

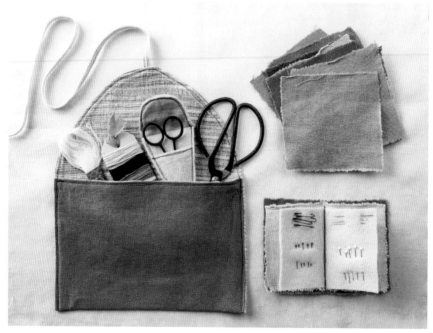

FLAX. Flax linen is one of our best options for a sustainable fiber, as it needs minimal water, fertilizer, and pesticides, it requires little energy to manufacture, and it can be composted at the end of its life.

HEMP. Growing hemp doesn't require the use of fertilizers or pesticides, and it can be made into a wide variety of fabrics, including canvas, denim, twill, jersey, and fleece.

LYOCELL. Commonly sold under the brand name Tencel, this fabric is made from wood pulp, typically eucalyptus wood, which grows quickly with little water and without pesticides. A particular spinning method allows the fabric to be naturally wrinkle resistant. Lyocell production does not create a lot of pollution, unlike its ugly cousin rayon. Viscose (aka rayon) can also be made from wood pulp but more often is made from petroleum, and toxic chemicals are used in its production. In fact, rayon workers sometimes develop cardiovascular and neurological health issues from exposure to the carbon disulfide used to make it.

SILK. Produced by caterpillars known as silkworms, this natural fabric is lightweight and durable. At the end of its life, it breaks down naturally. Commonly used for evening wear, it also makes surprisingly warm thermal underwear. Many ethical vegetarians avoid silk because producing it usually involves killing the silkworms. However, Peace Silk, also known as vegan silk, is a cruelty-free silk option.

WOOL. Wool is the hair or fur of sheep, goats, alpaca, and other animals. Animal fleece grows every year after shearing, so wool is considered a natural, renewable fiber source,

and a sustainable material. Many small wool producers are mindful of animal welfare and share details about their practices on their websites so you can research the quality of sources before purchase.

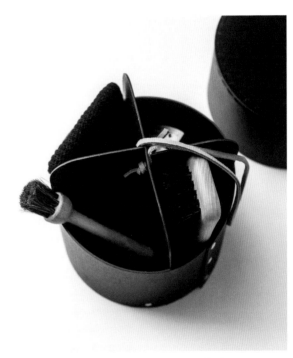

This shoeshine kit includes a shoe brush, dauber, cloth, and polish, all in sturdy cardboard with a convenient handle for easy transport.

FLEECE POLICE

The day I learned that fleece is made of plastic, and a huge contributor of microplastics in our environment, I had to rethink outdoor gear completely. I grew up in the Pacific Northwest, where we love clothes that allow us to venture out in any weather. But most clothing made for the outdoors is plastic. This is true for waterproof jackets, fleece, and stretchy items made for cycling, yoga, and running. I've made many trips to my favorite stores to look for nonplastic clothing and have found very few options. Even the high-end and well-made brands use highly toxic compounds of polytetrafluoroethylene (PTFE), the same chemical in Teflon. To avoid plastics and chemicals in sports clothes, be sure to check the labels and research each material.

Dust

Household dust is not as innocuous as it sounds. The higher the concentration of house dust, the more defensive our immune system gets, and a hyperalert immune system can cause a lot of health problems. Dust is made up of natural detritus from humans and pets, including skin cells, fur, and hair, as well as tiny particles from fabrics. It's filled with the same chemicals that contaminate our personal care products, clothing, and cookware, like perfluorooctanoic acid (PFOA) and BFRs. Some of these chemicals raise cholesterol levels, so removing dust can help reverse high cholesterol levels for many people. I've had clients with "stubborn cholesterol"—which is elevated cholesterol that doesn't come down with dietary changes—whose cholesterol levels dropped once they implemented the detox cleaning method and removed all the dust in their homes, much to their surprise and delight.

Since plastic is so prevalent in most homes, plastic particles are also common in dust, and we end up breathing them in. The phthalates these plastics contain are endocrine-disrupting chemicals that act like hormones in our bodies, sending erroneous messages to cells and confusing our hormone systems. As these nanoplastics make their way into our blood, they also become part of the plaque in our arteries. Perhaps the most surprising way that dust becomes highly toxic is that these plastic particles are superabsorbent; they act like sponges that hold on to a wide range of concerning chemicals.

You'll find some of the most chemically complex dust in the bedroom. Particulates from foam, pillows, and mattress material are released into the air and onto the floor, where they can become trapped in synthetic carpet fibers. On top of that, fibers from clothing, laden with formaldehyde and heavy metals, also become part of the dust.

Electronics

Electromagnetic fields (EMFs) are invisible waves of energy that have been proven to contribute to headaches, anxiety, and even tumor growth. There are four basic forms of EMFs.

MAGNETIC FIELDS surround any wire in which current is moving. They are also created by devices such as speakers and motors. The strength of a magnetic field decreases over distance.

ELECTRIC FIELDS emanate from wires that have electricity in use. They are attracted to conductors, like your body or metal.

RADIO FREQUENCY (RF) RADIATION is a higher-frequency transmission emitted from cell towers and radio station broadcast antennae. Gadgets like cell phones, routers, microwave ovens, and computers all use and emit RF radiation.

MICROSURGE ELECTRICAL POLLU-TION (MEP), also known as high-frequency voltage transients or dirty electricity, is the result of interference on electrical wires created by transformers, inverters, computers, and many other devices that use switch mode power supplies. MEP wave forms are similar to RF radiation, but they are in a frequency range that is particularly damaging to our biology, between 100 and 400 kilohertz.

The best way to reduce EMF exposure is to turn off your modem at night. Some modem boxes have an on/off switch, and some must be unplugged. I highly recommend removing electronic devices from the bedroom to reduce ambient light and EMFs. Removing electronics from the bedroom might seem odd at first, but once you get used to it, you might wonder why you ever created that chaos to begin with. Try it for a few weeks and experience the priceless psychological benefit of having the bedroom be a safe place for reading, cuddling, sex, talking, and rest. Banishing electronic devices from the bedroom can improve your sleep patterns and removes the temptation to look at your phone upon waking and being bombarded by the news or work email first thing in the morning. Give your whole family, including your pets, a break from the constant assault of EMFs and keep all electronics in your office or some other room where they can recharge at night. Use a battery-powered alarm clock; batteries do not emit EMFs, which makes them a safer option.

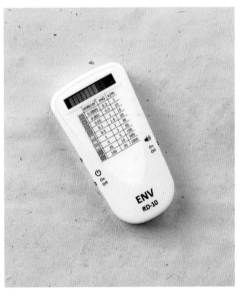

The ENV RD-10 is an easy-to-use meter to measure EMF hotspots around your home.

Mattresses

Mattresses are a primary source of toxins in the home. Synthetic mattresses are saturated with materials that have been linked to serious health complications, including polybrominated diphenyl ether (PBDE) and other flame-retardant chemicals that disrupt thyroid hormones. Flexible foam and memory foam mattresses off-gas high levels of VOCs that trigger airway inflammation and sleep apnea.

In addition, as we sleep, the heat, moisture, and movement from our bodies continually break down the foam, fabric, and synthetic rubber, causing the release of particles that become toxic dust. This causes secondary exposure through the dusty air that we breathe in our bedrooms.

Careful consideration of our mattress material is warranted because of the amount of time we spend sleeping and the close proximity of our faces to the material. Old synthetic mattresses can cause allergies, acne, eye mites, migraines, sinus inflammation, and asthma due to the release of contaminants. Over time, mattresses can become infested with bugs, bacteria, and fungus.

SYNTHETIC FOAM. You may have coil or synthetic foam mattresses that are decades old. These can fall apart as they age and release particulate matter as they deteriorate. New synthetic mattresses have other problems, including off-gassing and highly toxic synthetic foam made with flame retardants and chemicals intended to create a moisture barrier and reduce staining.

CASES AND COVERS. One way to salvage an old mattress is to cover it in a natural and nontoxic fabric mattress zipper encasement. These are made from cotton, and they rarely get washed because they are a bear to take off and require a large washing machine. Sturdy wool zipper cases work well to contain mattress materials, but they cannot be washed because they may shrink when drying, making them difficult to get back over the mattress.

If you use a zipper encasement, you will need an additional cotton topper that is washable to protect the mattress and its encasement. These are called mattress covers and look like heavy-duty fitted sheets. When shopping for covers, keep in mind that although it may be tempting to buy a plastic case because they are inexpensive, they should be avoided due to off-gassing and microplastic shedding. Also, avoid mattress covers that claim to be waterproof, as the waterproofing is achieved with synthetic material and chemicals like vinyl and PFOAs. Organic cotton covers hold up well in the wash and add a little extra cushion. These nontoxic cases and covers can minimize exposure to the chemicals embedded in your existing mattress. This is a great strategy if you're not ready to invest in a new natural material mattress.

NATURAL NONTOXIC LATEX. If you are ready for a new mattress, one of the best options is natural latex. They are sustainable and nontoxic as long as they are 100 percent natural latex rather than a combination of latex with synthetics. Synthetic latex is made from synthetic rubber, which is made from a variety of plastic polymers. Synthetic latex carries all the same risks as plastic in terms of phthalates, VOCs, and BFRs.

When shopping for latex mattresses, you will see the terms Dunlop and Talalay used to describe the latex. These are almost identical materials. Both are wonderful. They are both made from pure latex sap, tapped from beneath the bark of the rubber tree. The sap is harvested, whipped into a froth, and then set with natural agents like sulfur or zinc that turn liquid latex into a solid substance. The mattresses are made by baking sheets of latex foam in huge steam molds. The sheets of latex are stacked in layers inside a case of wool or cotton to create an all-natural mattress.

FUTON OR SHIKIBUTON. These are another good option. Made from wool and organic cotton, they are less expensive than latex. They are firm and offer great back support, but they don't have the bounce or spring of latex. If possible, shop for mattresses in person rather than online so you can test them yourself before purchasing.

• ● •

BEDBUG TREATMENT

Commercial bedbug treatments are very toxic. You can treat a bedbug infestation effectively with oregano or thyme essential oil. The two oils contain monoterpenoids (carvacrol in oregano, thymol in thyme) that have been proven effective in killing and repelling bedbugs.

½ cup water
1 tablespoon oregano or thyme essential oil

Combine the ingredients in a spray bottle and shake well. Mist all areas of the affected mattress with the spray. Open windows to ventilate the room, and let the mattress dry. Then vacuum thoroughly to remove dead bugs.

Memory Foam

Memory foam is everywhere these days; it is one of the most significant toxins in our homes. Most commercial memory foam mattress toppers are made of synthetic polyurethane that contains an incredible number of chemicals, including acetone, adhesives, antimony trioxide, benzene, diisocyanates, flame retardants (including PBDE), formaldehyde, heavy metals, isocyanates, lead, liquid carbon dioxide, mercury, methylene chloride, phthalates, polyester, roach killer, synthetic petroleum-based latex, toluene, and VOCs. This caustic cocktail can be especially health damaging for children, pets, and those who are immune compromised.

Mold

In bedrooms, as in bathrooms, elevated heat and moisture can encourage mold growth. Our bodies release a lot of heat and moisture at night as we breathe and sweat, and mold spores exist in all homes.

To keep mold under control in your bedroom, use a cloth with Tea Tree Spray to remove any visible mold from moist areas such as the base of the bed's headboard, around windows and windowsills, and on shelves and flooring, especially in closets or near heat sources. Ventilate your bedroom well by opening windows, running an air purifier, or turning on a fan.

REAL LIFE HOME DETOX
THE MEMORY FOAM PROBLEM

I worked with a couple in their mid-50s who both reported frequent headaches and feeling so tired it was as if they had been sedated. They were losing days of work due to the severity of their headaches, and the daily corticosteroids their doctor recommended were taking a toll on their bodies. They were highly motivated for a change. As I went through their house looking for possible triggers for their symptoms, I smelled something like chemicals in their bedroom. They explained that their mattress and most of their bedding were hand-me-downs from family members, except for a few memory-foam pillows and a memory-foam mattress topper. When I learned that they had been sleeping on memory foam, their symptoms were not as mysterious. Headaches, sinus pain, and fatigue are common reactions to polyurethane foam.

They agreed to purchase a natural latex mattress with a wool case in hopes of reducing their symptoms. Once the new natural mattress arrived, they found that they slept better than ever, their inflammation cleared up, they rarely experienced headaches, and no longer needed steroids. On a follow-up visit, I noticed that they both looked healthier and had less inflammation, and the bags under their eyes were reduced.

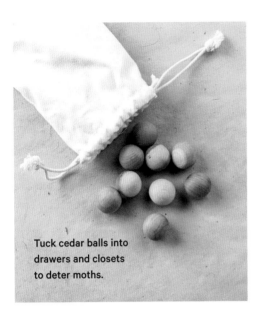

Tuck cedar balls into drawers and closets to deter moths.

Mothballs

First, moths are nothing to be feared. They are, after all, just gentle little flutter-bys. Of course, they can become an annoyance when their taste for wool and silk leaves holes in your wardrobe. Even so, moths can be easily removed and deterred from returning without the use of toxins.

Mothballs are overkill, a toxic holdover from the past that create a poisonous environment for humans and animals. Old anti-moth products, whether balls, cubes, spheres, cakes, powder, or flakes, are all the same combination of naphthalene and paradichlorobenzene (PDCB). Mothballs turn from a solid to vapor over time, which means they slowly release PDCB, a neurotoxin so powerful that it can damage the liver, kidneys, and lungs when ingested or inhaled. When pets or children ingest even small amounts, it can cause central nervous system toxicity and neurological damage.

Fortunately, there is no reason to bring this danger into the home. If you already have mothballs, wear gloves or use a disposable rag to pick them up, seal them in a leak-proof container, and toss them out. Then clean all the areas where you have seen moths. Clean hard surfaces where you store fabric, including closet floors, drawers, and shelves, with Tea Tree Wash, which will remove moth larvae. Wash clothing and fabrics to make them less attractive to moths, which mainly feed on natural materials that have some human sweat and microbe residue. Shake wool blankets and rugs outside and vacuum them well. Hang untreated cedar rings over hangers and put cedar balls in drawers, and add a few drops of cedar, clove, vetiver, or sandalwood essential oil to the cedar every few months to prevent moths from returning.

Pillows

We spend about a third of our lives sleeping, and our beds and pillows collect enormous amounts of living organisms, like mold, mites, and fleas, that trigger inflammation and infections. Given the time we spend sleeping and the proximity of the pillow to our airways, synthetic and feather pillows can be a primary trigger for ill health. This has important implications for people with respiratory disease, especially asthma and sinusitis. A study at the University of Manchester in the United Kingdom looked at synthetic and feather pillows used for periods ranging from a few months up to 20 years and found, on average, more than one million fungal spores in each pillow. The most common species were

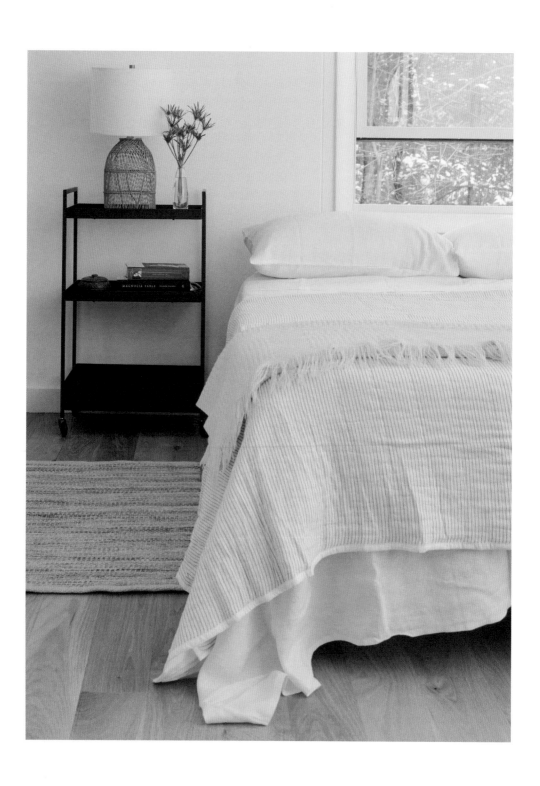

Aspergillus fumigatus, Aureobasidium pullulans, and *Rhodotorula mucilaginosa.* Another 47 species were found in pillows and vacuum dust. The number of species isolated per pillow varied from 4 to 16, with a higher number in synthetic pillows.

Beyond the danger from microbes, the materials that go into making pillows can be just as harmful. Polyurethane, commonly found in foam pillows, emits PBDE, which can cause thyroid dysfunction as well as foggy brain, acne, and fatigue. All the chemicals in memory foam mattresses are in memory foam pillows, too, and sleeping on them means hours of deep breathing these toxins into your lungs every night. There are several nontoxic, eco-conscious pillow options.

ORGANIC WOOL pillows are breathable, regulate temperature well, and are naturally mite resistant.

KAPOK is a fine, fibrous substance similar to cotton that grows around the seedpods of the ceiba (kapok) tree. It is used as stuffing for cushions, soft toys, and pillows. It is hypoallergenic, mold resistant, and quick drying.

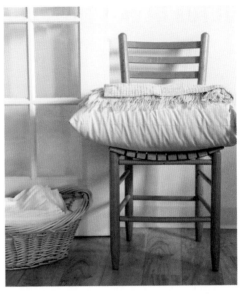

NATURAL LATEX is the milky sap from rubber trees. It is made into various density pillows, from soft to firm. It's hypoallergenic and lasts for years.

BUCKWHEAT pillows are filled with buckwheat hulls, which are hypoallergenic.

MILLET grain is dried and used as a hypoallergenic pillow filler material.

ORGANIC COTTON is used both to fill pillows and as pillowcases.

WHAT ARE OBESOGENS?

Obesogens are chemicals that interfere with the endocrine system and interrupt metabolism in ways that lead to an increase in body fat. Heavy metals and plastics—prevalent in synthetic mattresses, pillows, and other bedding—are obesogens. When you remove synthetic bedding and get proper REM sleep cycles, your endocrine system works better and helps boost your metabolism. By replacing bedding with natural materials and keeping your bedroom clean, you are more likely to have peaceful, regenerative sleep.

DETOX CLEAN THE BEDROOM

CLEANING YOUR BEDROOM involves a complete antibacterial surface cleanse, including getting rid of dust, which is, as we've discussed, a substantial carrier of toxins and pathogens. Use natural methods for each step, including essential oils rather than biocides for bedbugs, moths, and mold.

As you identify sources of potential toxins in your bedroom, you'll have to make decisions about what to do with them. Very few toxic items can be recycled. Synthetic fabrics and mattresses will have to be thrown out. But the most toxic items, like those containing memory foam, must be taken to a toxic waste facility.

Air

Open windows and turn on a fan to allow dust to escape as you clean.

Ceiling and Walls

Start by removing light fixtures, cleaning out bugs and dust, and cleaning the glass. Then dust around the ceiling, corners, and walls. If the walls are painted (rather than papered), spray them with Tea Tree Wash and wipe down with clean dry cloths, replacing the cloth often to avoid spreading dust.

Floor and Carpet

Vacuum carpets and floors thoroughly. Ventilate the room as you work by opening windows and doors and running a fan. Vacuum rugs or shake them outside. Wear a mask to protect yourself from dust.

Windows, Mirrors, and Picture Frames

If visible mold or moisture is collecting on the windows or sills, spray with Tea Tree Wash, dry thoroughly, and use a dehumidifier to remove the moisture in the air. Use Glass Spray to clean windows, the glass in picture frames, and mirrors.

Curtains and Blinds

Wash bedroom curtains as often as needed. If you have pets or smokers in the house, the curtains will likely need a monthly trip to the washing machine. If you locate mold anywhere in the room, wash the curtains with hot water, liquid soap, and 10 drops of tea tree essential oil. Dry the curtains thoroughly before rehanging them, as damp fabrics become a breeding ground for microbial growth.

If you have blinds or shutters, mist every surface with Tea Tree Wash and wipe down with a dry cloth to remove all particles of dust, microbes, and toxins.

Closet

Vacuum closets well, removing dust and cobwebs. Use Tea Tree Wash to clean hangers, shelves, and the floor. Wash any clothing that's soiled or that doesn't smell fresh, and make sure all clothes are dry before hanging them or tucking them back into drawers.

Bedding

Clean bed frames by misting with Tea Tree Wash and wiping down all surfaces. Wash sheets, mattress pads, blankets, and pillows with hot water, Liquid Laundry Soap (page 19), and 10 drops of tea tree essential oil. Dry all bedding thoroughly. When drying down pillows or blankets, consider using wool dryer balls to fluff them; they reduce clumping and drying time.

Drawers

Remove all items from each dresser and table drawer and spray the interior with Tea Tree Wash. Wipe out and let dry thoroughly before replacing items.

NICE GOING!

Take a few deep breaths. What a difference! Enjoy your fresh bed and truly clean bedroom. Rest easy knowing that the hours you are sleeping will be truly restorative.

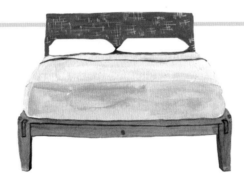

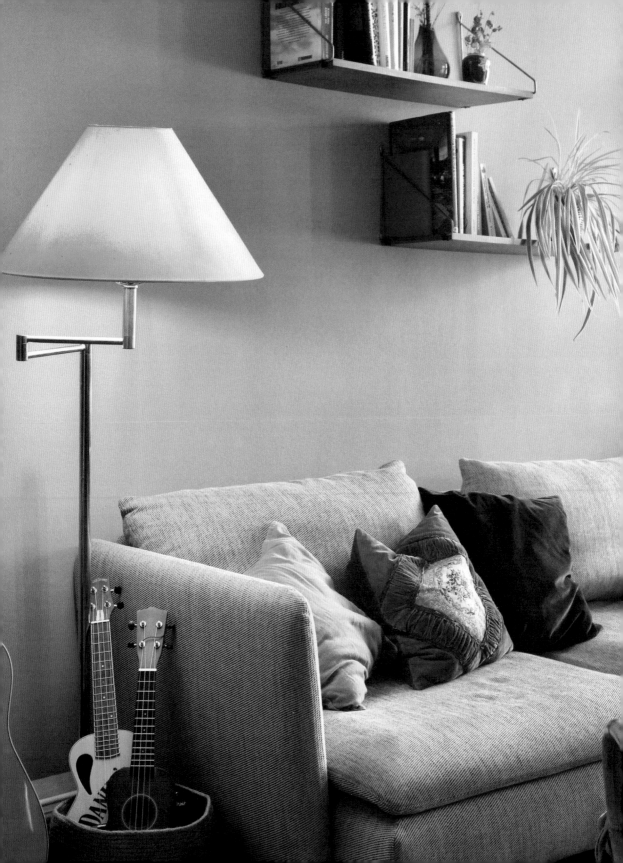

5
LIVING ROOM

Transforming the living room into a safe place to gather offers a high payoff for the work involved. We spend a lot of quality time in this space, listening to music, playing games, watching movies, and hanging out with each other. In my work helping people detoxify their homes, I have seen miraculous changes in the health of entire families and their pets when living room toxins are eliminated.

HIDDEN TOXINS IN THE LIVING ROOM

THE CLEANLINESS OF THE ROOM in which people gather and spend a lot of time—whether you call it the family room, TV room, or living room—will have a significant impact on your family's health. Pay close attention to the hang-out areas like the floor—where you might stretch out for yoga, where kids crawl around, where pets sleep—and the furniture you sink into to watch movies or read for hours.

Candles

Some candles are made of paraffin, which is a petroleum by-product, and older candles may have lead wicks, even though they have been banned in the US since 2003. Many candles also contain synthetic fragrances that emit VOCs that can irritate the eyes, skin, and lungs.

Look for beeswax candles as a nontoxic alternative. The downside is that they are more expensive than paraffin candles. In fact, many candle manufacturers blend paraffin with beeswax to cut costs; avoid these products and look for "100 percent beeswax" on labels.

Carpet

Wall-to-wall synthetic carpets are made stain resistant by being treated with per- and poly-fluoroalkyl substances (PFAS)—the same chemical used to make Teflon pans. These PFAS affect all living beings who are exposed to them. Toddlers and pets who spend time on the floor will have higher exposure. In addition, PFAS are "forever chemicals" meaning they don't break down under normal environmental conditions.

In addition to the PFAS, carpets also contain acetaldehyde, acetone, bromine, dyes, flame retardants, formaldehyde, glues, propanol, and VOCs.

When replacing carpet, consider wool, cork, tile, natural linoleum, or wood with a low VOC finish. If the floor covering needs an underlayment, consider wool padding and avoid polyurethane foam. Also avoid flooring that requires the use of synthetic glues to secure it; use nails or click-in flooring instead.

Natural-fiber rugs made from wool, jute, sisal, and organic cotton are inherently clean and generally free of stain-resistant treatments. High-quality rugs are worth the price. Buy them only from companies that provide clear information about the materials. Also, pay close attention to the materials in the rug backing and any pad you might use under it.

Curtains

Curtains retain airborne particles, such as dust, fireplace and candle smoke, and cleaning products. In homes where people smoke cigarettes, cadmium has been detected at high levels in the curtains. This heavy metal is linked to tumors in the kidneys, breast, and prostate. If you have curtains, make sure they can be machine washed so you can clean them regularly.

Make sure your curtains are made of natural fabric. Wood shutters and slats and pleated paper shades are other natural options. Check to be sure they are free of flame retardants, pesticides, PVC, glues, and foam.

TOXIC TEN

1. CANDLES
2. CARPET
3. CURTAINS
4. DÉCOR
5. ELECTRONICS
6. FIREPLACE
7. INCENSE
8. LEATHER
9. UPHOLSTERY
10. WOOD FURNITURE

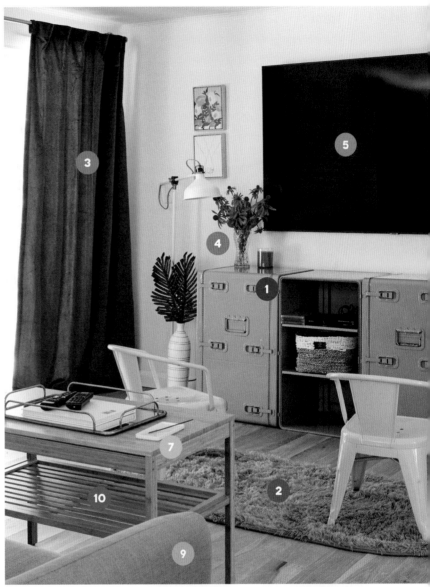

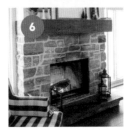

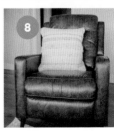

Décor

Our decorations or ornamentations all collect dust and require frequent cleaning. And the more items in a home, the more likely it is that toxic materials have been brought in with them. Many metal objects contain lead, many fake flowers are made of plastic, and plush toys are stuffed with toxic foam. Over time, as we've seen with all household items, they release small particles of these materials into the air, and either we breathe them in, or eventually they fall to the floor and become toxic components of the household dust.

The more objects in a room, the longer it will take to clean. First you have to clear surfaces in order to clean them; then you have to clean the items you just cleared. The longer I've been steeped in this research, the simpler my home has become. I find that minimalism has many benefits. It feels surprisingly relaxing to have fewer objects around. I don't have to worry about the potential health risks of objects, and I have fewer things to clean.

Electronics

Concerns about electronics in the living room begin with electromagnetic fields (EMFs). EMFs affect the nervous system of all mammals, like humans and our pets, interfering with the communication between cells. Scientists have also found a clear connection between residential exposure to extremely low-frequency magnetic fields (ELFs) and childhood leukemia. If you test the electronics in your home with an EMF meter, as I did, it becomes clear that EMFs stay close to the device that emits them. When you move back just a few feet from the television,

for example, EMF levels drop off. Most adults sit far enough away from televisions and screens, but children tend to like to be right in front of them. Creating seating for kids that is at least three feet from large screens will help reduce their exposure.

The plastic casings on most electronics, like computer monitors and especially TVs, are made with high levels of brominated flame retardants (BFRs). In fact, flame retardants can make up between 1 and 33 percent of the weight of TV enclosures.

It is possible to find TVs that are BFR-free. Toxic-Free Future tested top brands of televisions for BFR levels and published a list (available online) of those with the lowest levels. However, the organization found only one TV that was free of all flame retardants.

Fireplace

The smoke from wood burning is made up of a complex mixture of gases and fine particles. These microscopic particles can get into eyes and the respiratory system, causing your eyes to burn and your nose to run and potentially triggering asthma, bronchitis, and migraines. In addition, wood smoke contains several toxic air pollutants including acrolein, benzene, formaldehyde, and PAHs. PAHs act as free radicals; they are particularly harmful to people with suppressed immune systems.

If you use a fireplace in your home, it's important that it vents effectively. Make sure the chimney is clear of obstruction, which will likely require a professional service. Call a chimney sweep service to learn more about your fireplace's maintenance needs.

Incense

Incense is a supertoxin! Given the same duration of exposure, burning incense is more toxic to cells and carries a higher risk for causing cancer than smoking cigarettes. It releases dangerous pollutants into the house, including carbon monoxide, PAHs, and VOCs.

Smoke from incense causes inflammation in the lungs and liver, oxidative stress, and asthmatic symptoms. It contains a multitude of well-studied carcinogens, and long-term exposure to the smoke is associated with an increased risk of squamous cell carcinoma of the respiratory tract. A recent study found that a particular compound released when incense is burned, auramine O (AuO), promotes the growth of lung tumor cells. And studies with children found that daily exposure to burning incense is associated with impaired adolescent lung function.

Sometimes people burn incense to cover up a bad smell. In this case, deep cleaning and possibly repairing bigger issues, like water damage that's led to the growth of mold, could be the answer. If your home is clean, then opening windows for fresh airflow should be adequate for getting rid of residual smells from cooking or dogs, for example. For around-the-clock air purification, air-purifying houseplants are your best bet (see page 128). If you're looking to add fragrance, try misting with an Essential Oil Spritzer (page 18) or, occasionally, burning naturally aromatic leaves, such as dried sage.

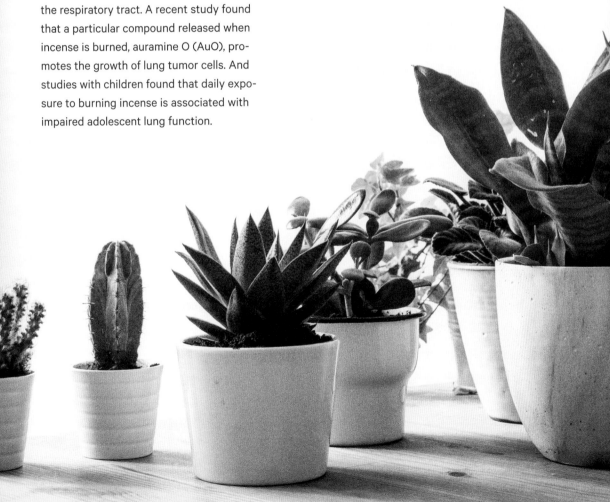

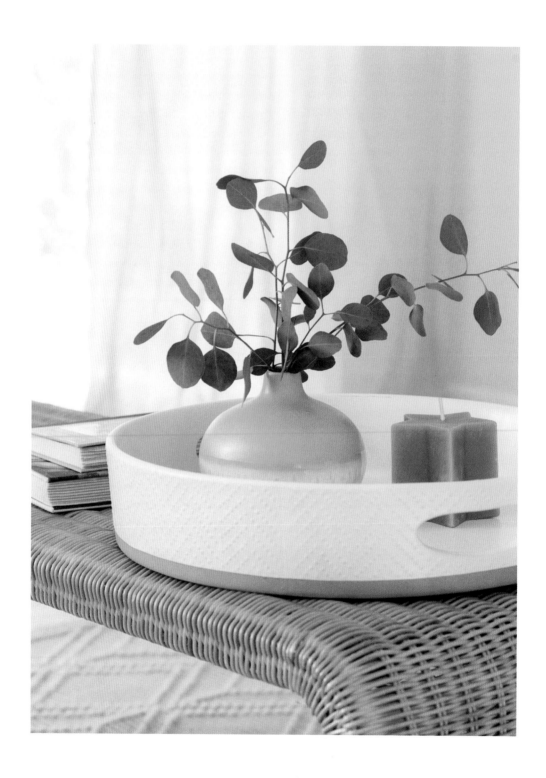

Leather

Many leather items are treated with a toxic slush of chromium salts and tanning materials that produce a supple and richly colored look but are also highly carcinogenic. Some of the glues used to process leather create VOCs from methylene chloride and ethyl acetate, as well as formaldehyde. Per- and polyfluoroalkyl substances (PFAS), the same compounds used in Teflon pans, are also used to process some leather. Children exposed to these endocrine disruptors have been found to have an increased risk of obesity later in life, because they can trigger epigenetic changes that reduce the ability of cells to make energy and burn body fat.

Fake leather is generally made of synthetic materials like plastic. However, exciting new leather alternatives are being developed: washable paper leather, pineapple leather, and even mushroom leather (sometimes called mycelium leather).

Upholstery

The padding used for upholstered furniture—sofas, bench cushions, window cushions, decorative pillows, ottomans, and outdoor furniture cushions—is made of the same hazardous materials as mattresses. This polyurethane foam is treated with flame-retardant chemicals that off-gas and shed toxic foam particles for many years, which creates toxic dust and fumes in the air we breathe. We end up with so much in our bodies that flame retardants even show up in blood tests. In addition, stain guard–treated upholstery is coated in PFAS that emit into our homes for years.

Furniture stores are moving toward offering sustainable and nontoxic furniture, and material details are usually available online. If you already have upholstered furniture, clean your home often to remove dust and reduce your exposure. Avoid using after-market treatments like stain repellent sprays.

When you're buying new furniture, ask that the distributor skip the application of stain repellent and antimicrobial treatments, as they are toxic. Look for companies with ethical practices, such as repurposing discarded materials and using only Forest Stewardship Council (FSC) certified wood. Some companies offer levels of sustainability in the options for each layer of your furniture, such as using Dunlop latex or wool fill and 100 percent organic fabrics and ticking.

Wood Furniture

Wood seems like a naturally sustainable and nontoxic choice, but much of the new and popular furniture sold through large chain stores uses quick-and-dirty methods of production involving surface treatments and glues that release VOCs, such as benzene, ethyl acetate, toluene, and xylene.

One sustainable method for obtaining wood furniture is to seek out vintage or secondhand wood furniture. This avoids the harvest of trees (deforestation), and if you're lucky enough to get true vintage furniture it will likely have been crafted before the era of toxic glues.

If you're buying new wood furniture, avoid particleboard and other "pressed wood" products. Look for solid untreated wood that is free of synthetic chemicals.

DETOX CLEAN THE LIVING ROOM

THE INITIAL DEEP CLEANING of the living room can take significant time to remove toxic buildup from this frequently used space. After the first deep cleaning, you will find that this space will be much easier to maintain as many of the jobs may only need to be done annually, such as cleaning the carpets and the chimney.

Air

Open windows to ventilate the room as you clean.

Ceiling and Walls

Start high and work down. Remove light fixtures, clean out bugs and dust, and clean the glass. Dust, using a pole duster if needed to reach high ceilings, and clean the tops of any shelves and cabinets. If the walls are painted (rather than papered), spray them with Tea Tree Wash (page 21) and wipe down with a clean dry cloth, replacing the cloth often to avoid spreading dust.

Fireplace

Tackle the messy job of cleaning out the fireplace. If your fireplace burns wood, removing the ashes will improve airflow and help the wood burn more cleanly without as much smoke. Vacuum around the fireplace to clean up any spilled ashes or soot. Use a damp cloth to remove any ash dust left around the fireplace. If used often, the chimney will need to be cleaned about once a year to remove any blockages.

Furniture

Wipe down hard surfaces, such as coffee tables and wood chairs, with Tea Tree Wash. Remove cushions and vacuum sofas and upholstered furniture thoroughly.

Curtains and Blinds

Wash living room curtains as often as needed. If you have pets or smokers in the house, the curtains will likely need a monthly trip to the washing machine. If you locate mold anywhere in the room, wash the curtains with hot water, liquid soap, and 10 drops of tea tree essential oil. Dry the curtains thoroughly before rehanging them, as damp fabrics become a breeding ground for microbial growth.

If you have blinds or shutters, mist every surface with Tea Tree Wash and wipe down with a dry cloth to remove all particles of dust, microbes, and toxins.

Carpets

If you have synthetic carpets, use a steamer, which you can usually rent from a hardware store, to clean them. Help them dry thoroughly by turning up the heat. Crack open windows to let out the moisture and to ventilate fumes. Once the carpets are clean, consider a no-shoes policy in the house. Also think about replacing any synthetic carpets with natural materials, such as wool.

Floors

Vacuum floors thoroughly, then spray with Tea Tree Wash and wipe dry with a clean cloth to disinfect and remove dust and grime. If the floor is vinyl or tile, you may need to use Tub Scrub (page 21) to remove debris and scrub away layers of previously used cleaning products.

WAY TO GO!

Take a few deep breaths. You have dramatically reduced the health risks in your living room. Enjoy the fresh air, cozy seating, and truly clean floors as you socialize, play games, watch movies, and read.

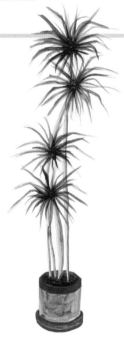

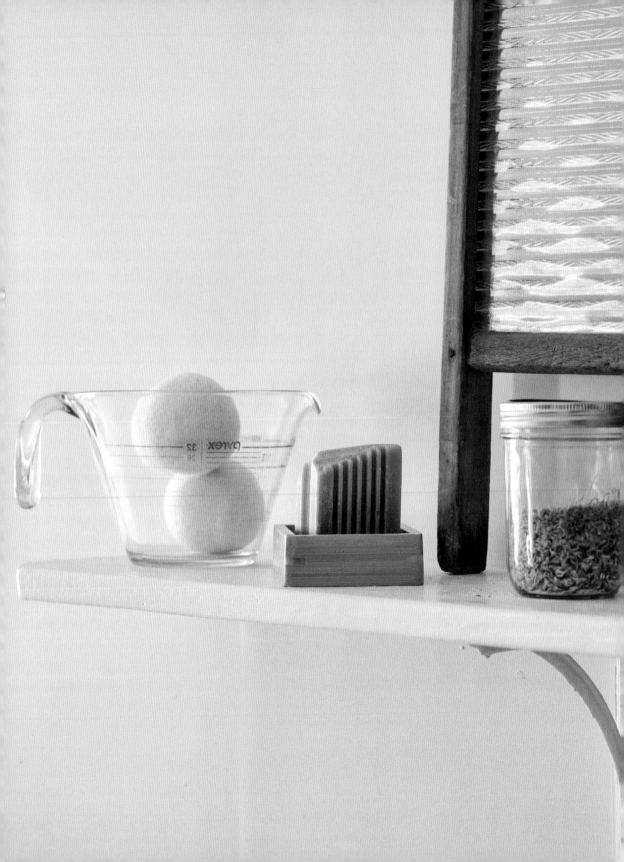

6
LAUNDRY ROOM

Making changes in your laundry habits is one of the most impactful ways to help the environment because we buy more laundry products than any other cleaning product and they can be downright poisonous. There are thousands of laundry products on store shelves, and almost every one of them contains VOCs that spread in the air throughout the house. Detoxing your laundry room is largely a matter of reducing the number and toxicity of the products there.

HIDDEN TOXINS IN THE LAUNDRY ROOM

READ THE LABELS and you will find a shocking number of toxic chemicals in most laundry products. Even more concerning, when researchers tested common brands, they found hundreds of toxic compounds that were not disclosed on the product labels. Ingredients include surfactants like alkylbenzene sulfonates, quaternary ammonium compounds, alkylphenol ethoxylates, and alcohol ethoxylates that are not only toxic to humans but contaminate aquatic and land environments.

Laundry products can act as lung irritants that trigger asthma, allergies, and migraines. With asthma affecting nearly 1 in 10 American children, 26 million adults diagnosed with chemical sensitivity, and nearly 25 percent of households having someone who suffers from migraines, it makes sense to avoid exposure to known triggers.

A ridiculous number of laundry products are marketed to people every year, creating more plastic waste. The truth is, we don't need these products. Shop at your local co-op for clean and minimal-waste options. Most co-ops sell powdered and liquid laundry soap in bulk form, so you can bring your own container and skip the packaging altogether. Beware of "green-washing" in the household product aisles of mainstream stores. Even products that claim to be eco-friendly contain toxic chemicals. If a product contains words you don't know, don't buy it until you look them up. Making your own laundry cleaning supplies is easy, safe, inexpensive, and the best choice environmentally. You need only a few basic and safe ingredients, like Dr. Bronner's Sal Suds, washing soda, and dryer balls, to properly clean laundry.

Antistatic Spray

This unnecessary product is so toxic that you have to read a long list of first-aid measures in case you inhale it, ingest it, or get it on your skin or in your eyes. These sprays contain propellants that cause skin and eye irritation, quaternary ammonium compounds, and synthetic fragrances.

Wool dryer balls can replace antistatic spray and last for years. Every laundry room should have them. For extreme cases of static cling, a mist of water will solve the problem.

Bleach

Liquid chlorine bleach is sodium hypochlorite, which can be an irritant in dilute amounts and deadly when concentrated. Also, using this laundry bleaching product may create chlorinated by-products, many of which are cancer-causing compounds. Chlorine is volatile and should never be combined with anything else, even natural materials. For example, combining it with vinegar or other acids will create highly toxic chlorine gas, which can cause severe burns internally and externally. Worst of all, mixing bleach with ammonia produces toxic chloramine gas.

Bleach is toxic and unnecessary. There are many effective fabric-lightening alternatives, including baking soda, lemon juice, and vinegar. Each of these natural cleaners is safe and inert.

TOXIC TEN

1. ANTISTATIC SPRAY
2. BLEACH
3. DRYER LINT
4. DRYER SHEETS
5. DRYER VENTS
6. FABRIC SOFTENER
7. LAUNDRY DETERGENT
8. LAUNDRY PODS
9. MOLD AND MILDEW
10. STAIN REMOVER

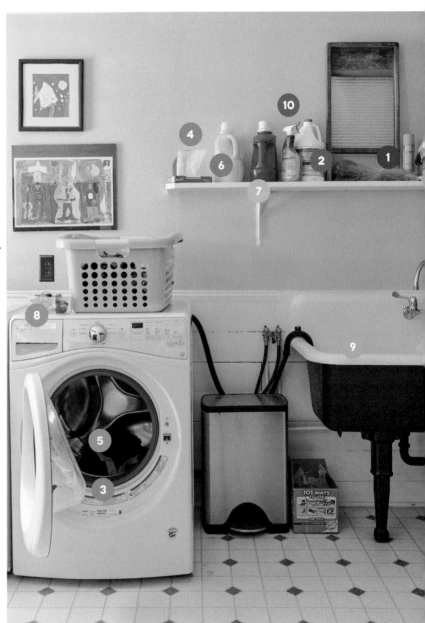

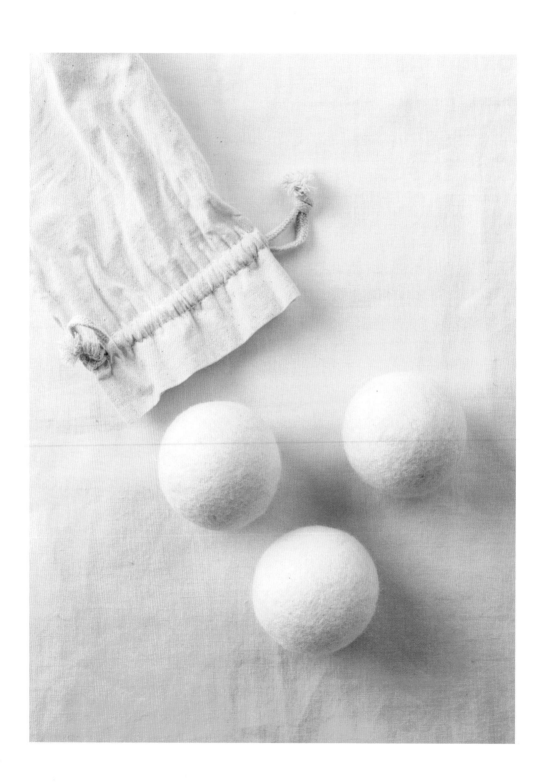

Dryer Lint

Every time we use a dryer, some of the lint ends up in the air in the laundry room, and as airborne dust, it carries chemicals from laundry products and microbes throughout the house. Lint from synthetic materials like fleece, microfiber, and spandex contains high levels of chemicals such as polybrominated diphenyl ethers and phthalate esters that end up in the air we breathe and the dust in our homes. These compounds also end up in our water systems and oceans.

Reduce toxic lint by cleaning the dryer screen after every load, switching to natural-fabric clothing, and using only environmentally friendly laundry products.

Dryer Sheets

Dryer sheets soften your clothes, but they are also supertoxins due to their level of solvents, synthetic fragrances, and VOCs.

Fragranced products like dryer sheets release chemicals into the air we breathe and onto the clothes we wear. These chemical fragrances also travel throughout the house, attaching to carpeting, curtains, and walls, creating a toxic film on surfaces. Most contain acetaldehyde, acetone, benzene, ethanol, and a whole slew of VOCs, some of which are classified as hazardous air pollutants by the EPA.

If you want to add fragrance to your laundry, you can do so safely by adding a few drops of essential oils to wool dryer balls, which are natural and nontoxic.

Dryers

A dryer is basically a box that heats air, tumbles clothes, and blows moist air through a hose so it can vent through a wall to the outside. If your dryer runs on gas rather than electricity, there is waste gas in the form of carbon monoxide (CO), which is colorless, odorless, and tasteless. CO is highly toxic and can be lethal. Symptoms of exposure include dull headache, chest pain, upset stomach, vomiting, fatigue, dizziness, and confusion. If the gas can't vent due to a kinked hose, blockage from lint buildup, or obstruction by a bird's nest, for example, the gas can flow back inside the house. Crack open a window to vent trapped gases and install a carbon monoxide alarm.

You can avoid this danger by air-drying your clothes on a line outside in the sun or on folding racks inside. When the racks are not in use, find a place to tuck them away or add a couple of hooks to the wall to hang them so they're not underfoot.

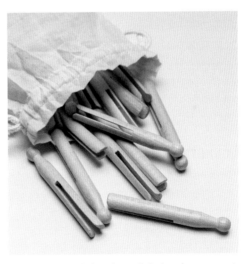

Strong and sturdy beechwood clothespins are great for use indoors or outdoors. The biodegradable pegs come in a cloth bag for easy storage, and they don't rust, so they don't leave stains on clothes.

A MYSTERIOUS ILLNESS

A client called because he was having stomach issues and cognitive problems, including poor memory and trouble putting his thoughts together. He spent his mornings shoveling snow, and when he reported to me that he felt better when he was working outside than when at home, I knew he needed to have his home checked for toxins. He brought in a contractor, who immediately noticed that the dryer vented directly into his house. He was being poisoned around the clock because the dryer was running most of the time to dry out his wet work clothes and wet dog bedding. The contractor was able to create a proper venting system, and my client immediately started to feel better. His story ended well, but I have to wonder how many others are exposed to carbon monoxide; there are many sources in the home, including water heaters, furnaces, gas- and wood-burning fireplaces, and gas stoves and ovens.

Fabric Softener

Fabric softener is one of those products that no one needs. It's just one more chemical cocktail in a plastic bottle. Americans spend $700 million a year keeping their fabrics soft by coating them with chemicals.

Use wool dryer balls instead. They work wonders as they gently bounce around, fluffing and softening fabrics naturally. They also shorten drying time considerably.

Laundry Detergent

There are hundreds of laundry detergents on the market, and almost all of them are completely synthetic and contain long lists of dangerous chemicals, including chlorine bleach, dioxane, formaldehyde, naphthas, phenols, phosphates, quaternary ammonium compounds, sodium borate, and synthetic fragrance.

Instead, look for products with recognizable, natural ingredients such as Castile soap, coconut oil, sodium bicarbonate (baking soda), sodium carbonate (washing soda), essential oils, and salt. It's also easy to make your own laundry soap (see page 19). Avoiding toxic laundry detergents not only protects you from hazardous exposures but also helps reduce plastic waste.

Laundry Pods

Laundry detergent capsules known as pods are a fairly new item on supermarket shelves. They are shiny and colorful and look a bit like candy; children have eaten them, causing severe reactions ranging from airway inflammation to esophageal perforation. They are very dangerous for children and pets and leave a significant toxic residue on fabrics. For these reasons, avoid laundry pods, and use natural laundry detergent or make your own instead.

Mold and Mildew

The humid environment in the laundry area encourages mildew growth. Cleaning around the washer and dryer, windows, and corners of the floor will help reduce the chances of mildew growth. There are several ways to reduce the chance of mildew growth in the laundry area.

DO LAUNDRY FREQUENTLY. A pile of damp clothes attracts mildew.

MOVE LAUNDRY FROM THE WASHER to the dryer as soon as it's done. Wet laundry grows mildew surprisingly fast and then gives off a telltale musty odor that stays with the fabrics even after they are dried.

LEAVE THE WASHER LID OPEN when it's not in use to allow the interior surfaces to dry.

REMOVE LINT FROM DRYER FILTERS for proper airflow to allow moisture to escape.

OPEN A WINDOW, run a fan, or use a dehumidifier to reduce humidity in your laundry room.

Stain Remover

The big picture here is that having spotless clothes at the expense of our health and the environment is a losing game. Stain remover is another unnecessary and highly risky product. Common toxins in stain removers include alkylbenzene sulfonate, butoxyethanol, quaternary ammonium compounds, sodium hypochlorite (chlorine bleach), and sodium borate (borax).

We rely too heavily on chemicals to do jobs that can be done with a tiny bit of effort. Simply soaking and spot scrubbing clothes will remove many stains. Try a little baking soda on fresh oil-based stains, or a drop of Castile soap and water on your next stubborn stain. Soak, scrub the spot, and then rinse well.

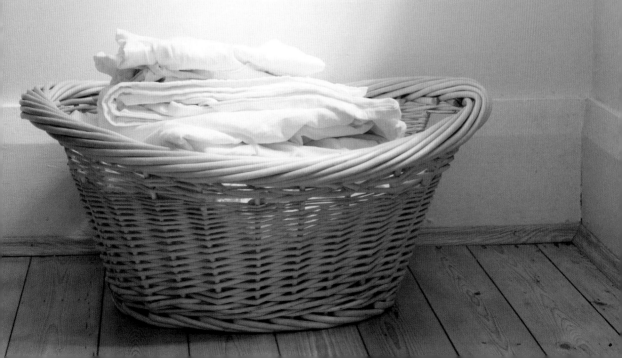

DETOX CLEAN THE LAUNDRY ROOM

LAUNDRY AREAS GET HEAVY USE, so set yours up to make it easy to use the space. A clean and organized laundry room makes laundering more enjoyable and less of a chore.

Air

Open a window or turn on a fan if you have one. This will help ventilate the room as you clean so you won't breathe in dust. Air circulation will also help the surfaces dry after you clean.

Ceiling and Walls

Start high and work down. Remove light fixtures, clean out bugs and dust, and clean the glass. Dust, using a pole duster if needed to reach high ceilings. Vacuum behind the washer and dryer. Laundry rooms have notoriously dirty walls. If the walls are painted (rather than papered), spray them with Tea Tree Wash (page 21) and wipe down with a clean dry cloth, replacing the cloth often to avoid spreading dust.

Dryer Vent

Check your vent regularly. Step outside the house to the vent outlet while the dryer is running to make sure the warm air from the dryer is flowing out easily. Clean out any visible lint in the vent from the outside. Back inside, also check behind the dryer to make the sure the outflow hose isn't kinked or broken. If you see cracks in the hose, replace it; if you can't replace it right away, seal the hose with duct tape. Make sure the hose is firmly attached to the dryer and the vent to the outside. Remove dryer lint from the mesh screen inside the dryer (the lint trap) before each use.

Shelves

Once you have removed and properly disposed of all the toxic products, use Tea Tree Wash to wipe down each shelf. Organize your nontoxic cleaning supplies so they are easy to reach. Keep wool dryer balls in a bowl or simply leave them in the dryer after each use.

Windows

When glass cools on one side and heats up on the other, condensation happens, and the area around the window is the most likely area for mildew formation. Mist Tea Tree Wash on the windowsill and around the glass where it meets the window frame to kill mildew and wipe the glass and surrounding area well with clean dry rags. Then clean windows with Glass Spray (page 18) and clean rags.

THAT'S QUITE AN IMPROVEMENT!

By removing the dust and mold, making repairs, and setting yourself up with non-toxic laundry products, you will have everything you need to make doing laundry a breeze. Enjoy your fresh work area and your truly clean laundry.

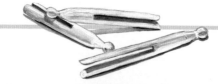

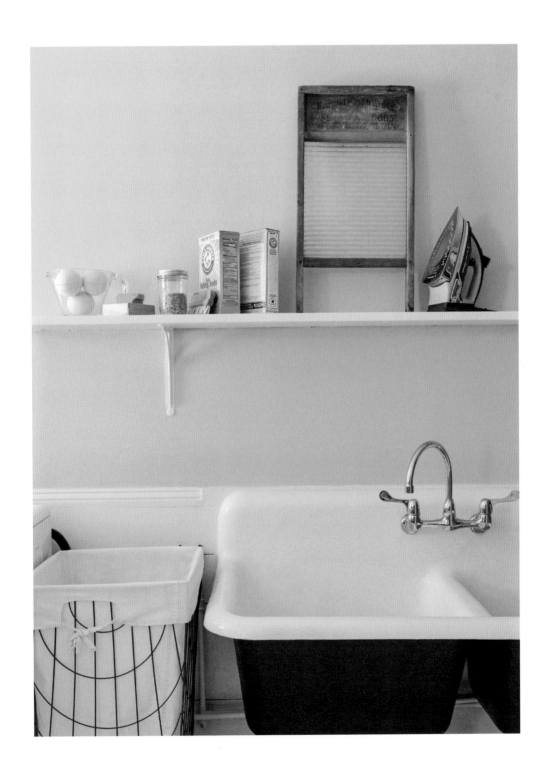

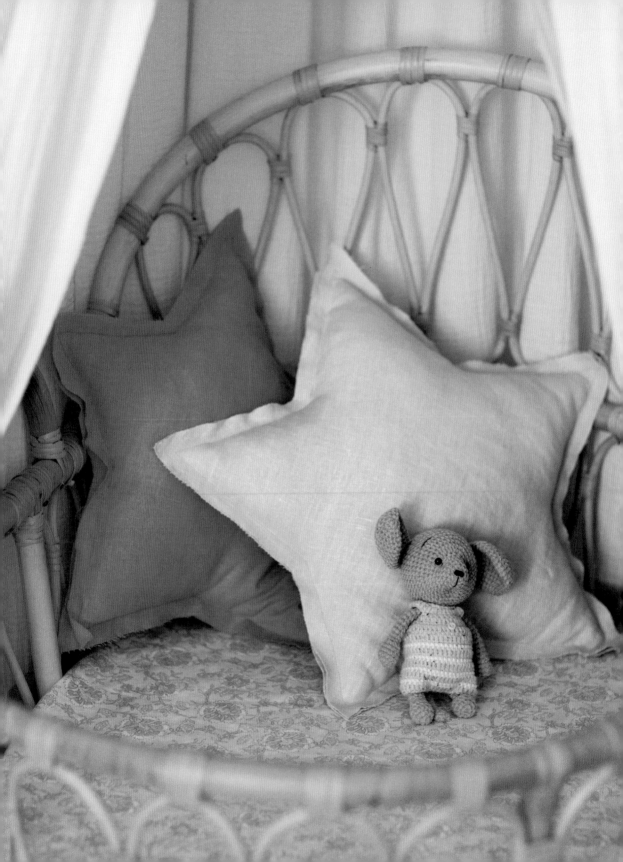

7

KIDS' ROOMS

Kids' rooms carry more risks due to the number of items and toys. An informed eye can review items in these rooms and consider replacing or refreshing mattresses, bedding, clothes, and toys. After removing and replacing items, you can home in on hidden toxic residues. Children spend a lot of time in their rooms, so it's important to reduce their exposure to airborne and contact toxins in this space.

HIDDEN TOXINS IN KIDS' ROOMS

CHILDREN ARE DISPROPORTIONATELY affected by toxic exposures due to their small size, which means a greater impact on their health. We will consider the number of plastic toys in kids' rooms, and assess flame retardants in items such as pajamas, sleeping bags, and mattresses. The goal is to reduce and avoid bringing into the room items that off-gas, including furniture, rugs, and paint, and eliminate electromagnetic field (EMF) exposures from electronics.

Baby Monitors

Many baby monitors, particularly wireless monitors and those with video monitoring, emit EMF radiation. This is concerning for a few reasons. First, this radiation source is often near newborn babies' heads all night, and their soft skulls allow deeper penetration of electromagnetic energy. Also, the collective and chronic exposure from electronics and their EMF emissions are suspected of causing epigenetic changes and increasing the risk for cancer. If you are using a baby monitor, be sure to keep it a minimum of four feet from a baby's crib.

Baby Skin Care Products

Hundreds of synthetic ingredients are added to baby skin care products to provide a pleasant scent, but many are respiratory irritants and sensitizers. These products contain the same harmful ingredients as adult skin care products, including parabens, synthetic fragrances, and alcohol. Oddly, baby products labeled as gentle, organic, fragrance-free, or designed for sensitive skin appear to contain as many allergens as those not marketed as such. The lesson here is that it is much safer to avoid commercial baby products altogether due to their toxic ingredients and a lack of regulation. Many baby products are unnecessary; there are healthy children all over the planet in areas without these products.

The skin readily absorbs whatever chemicals you put on it, so a good rule of thumb is that if you wouldn't eat it, don't put it on your baby's skin. Use only whole-plant ingredients such as jojoba oil, coconut oil, and almond oil on babies.

EXPOSURE THROUGH MOTHER'S COSMETICS

A large-scale study found that more than four million women are exposed daily to personal care product ingredients that are reproductive and developmental toxins, linked to impaired fertility or developmental harm for a baby in the womb or nursing.

TOXIC TEN

1. **BABY MONITORS**
2. **BABY SKIN CARE PRODUCTS**
3. **BASSINETS AND CRIBS**
4. **BOTTLES AND PACIFIERS**
5. **CARPET**
6. **CLOTHES**
7. **DIAPERS**
8. **ELECTRONICS**
9. **MATTRESSES**
10. **TOYS**

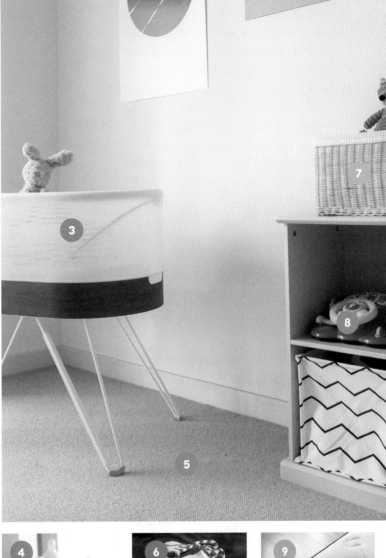

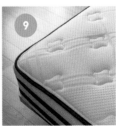

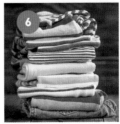

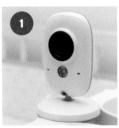

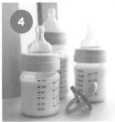

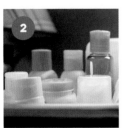

Bassinets and Cribs

Bassinets and cribs are often made with materials like plywood, pressed wood, particleboard, chipboard, or fiberboards that contain glues and plastics and may be finished with varnishes and paints that all carry risks for babies. Some of the most concerning contaminants found in new furniture made for babies include phthalates, triclosan, PFAs, and flame retardants. Solid wood bassinets and cribs are safer options. Look for nontoxic finishes, with certified safety levels such as GreenGuard Gold certification (see page 74).

Bottles and Pacifiers

Children are exposed to phthalates from many sources, including bottles, bottle nipples, and pacifiers, as well as toys, mattresses, food packaging, and food storage containers. It is estimated that the average adult intake of

plastic is 5 grams every week—and babies who are drinking through plastic nipples and chewing on plastic pacifiers take in even more.

Phthalate exposure is risky for children and babies. Some phthalates are associated with specific health risks such as exposure to dibutyl phthalate and benzyl butyl phthalate (BBP), which are linked to language delay in children. A common phthalate, di(2-ethylhexyl) phthalate (DEHP), that is in products like shower curtains, food packaging, and lunch boxes, has been found to be the largest contributor of phthalates. Infants and toddlers ingest DEHP via breast milk (due to the mother's exposure) as well as mouthing behavior. Avoid plastic and synthetic latex baby items whenever possible. Many companies now make baby items including nipples, pacifiers, and sippy cups in nontoxic materials such as silicone and 100 percent natural latex.

Carpet

It must have sounded like a great idea when someone first thought of using PFAS to make carpets stain resistant, but when children play on chemically treated carpets, they breathe in these chemicals and absorb them through their skin. Carpeting also holds on to pesticides and herbicides that are tracked in on shoes. When there are children in the house, a no-shoes policy mitigates risk and makes cleaning easier.

Hardwood and bamboo floors installed without glues are a couple of nontoxic flooring options. Wood floors won't collect and hold on to dust the way carpet does, and smooth floors can be cleaned well. Natural wool carpets without PFAS treatments are also an option.

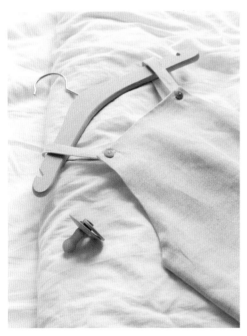

Clothing made of natural materials without the use of synthetic dyes, printing, or plastics reduces the risk of exposure to heavy metals, formaldehyde, and phthalates.

Clothes

Mass-produced children's clothing can contain any number of poisonous compounds, including synthetic dyes, phthalates, flame retardants, and formaldehyde. Kids' clothing with dyed fabrics and printed graphics were found to contain especially high concentrations of toxins, including chromium, copper, and lead; these metals are used to impart color.

Hand-me-downs are much less likely to contain metals and chemicals because most of the toxins are removed slowly over time from washings. When buying new clothes for children, avoid synthetic fabrics and dyes, and look for natural organic fabrics, with natural plant dyes. See the list of recommended fabrics on page 78.

Diapers

There is no doubt that disposable diapers are convenient, but are they safe? There are concerns. Disposable diapers are made of plastic and can contain methylene chloride, phthalates, polyethylene, polypropylene, synthetic dyes and fragrances, toluene, and xylene, among other toxins.

These chemicals are key factors in everything from chronic diaper rash to respiratory issues, male infertility, and testicular cancer. Although the risks have been well studied, most parents are not aware of the adverse effects of these products on babies' reproductive organs. Diaper dermatitis is a common problem reported by pediatricians, and it is linked to the various blue, pink, and green dyes in disposable diapers. Since disposable diapers are worn 24 hours a day for more than 2 years, the potential harm is significant.

Disposable diapers carry too many risks to be worth the convenience. Use 100 percent organic cotton cloth diapers instead. A diaper cleaning service can help make the transition to cloth much smoother. Keep a stack of washcloths and water with your changing area as an easy substitution for wipes.

Electronics

Protect kids from EMF exposure by removing all electronics from their rooms, including baby monitors, gaming devices, tablets, and televisions. Keep children away from electronics as much as possible. Children absorb more microwave radiation than adults because their brain tissues are more absorbent and their skulls are thinner. Many countries with technologically sophisticated governments are working to limit children's exposure to Wi-Fi and wireless devices, including Belgium, France, Germany, and India.

Limiting screen time is equally important. Creating distance from electronic devices also reduces exposure.

Mattresses

Many of the mattress issues discussed in the bedroom chapter (page 73) apply to crib and toddler bedding. Mattresses sold for cribs are notorious for their high toxin emissions. Infants spend most of their time sleeping, which exposes them to mattress materials for many hours a day. As they sleep, they are breathing in and ingesting mattress materials. The chemical emissions released from polyurethane foam and polyester crib mattress padding include flame retardants, waterproofing chemicals, and dozens of VOCs. This cocktail of chemicals created by baby bedding has been linked to sudden infant death syndrome (SIDS).

Children's bedding and mattresses contain so many toxic compounds that certifications have been developed to help consumers understand which products are safer. The Made Safe organization, for example, screens for behavioral toxins, carcinogens, developmental toxins, endocrine disruptors, heavy metal neurotoxins, high-risk pesticides, reproductive toxins, toxic solvents, and VOCs.

Look for nontoxic mattresses that are made from 100 percent natural latex rubber, organic cotton, wool, bamboo, or hemp.

CRIB MATTRESS COVERS. The plastic covers used to protect crib mattresses emit highly toxic gases, and a baby's body heat can increase the concentration of these gases. When tested, plastic gases were found to be about four times higher in the crib area than in the rest of the room. This elevates the baby's level of exposure to two dangerous compounds: DEHP and diisononyl phthalate (DINP), which cause liver, spleen, and kidney tumors, lower IQ, disrupt the endocrine system, and lead to airway inflammation so severe that it restricts oxygen to the baby. Avoid synthetic crib covers. Look for organic cotton covers, wool moisture pads, organic bamboo fitted crib mattress protectors, and the GOTS approval to ensure organic certification.

BEST BEDDING MATERIALS. Rather than try to make sense of all the materials used in babies' and children's mattresses and bedding, a much better strategy is to avoid all synthetics and opt for all-natural materials like breathable, 100 percent organic cotton and linen blankets and a latex rubber mattress. Look for stitching in the mattress, which indicates that glues and adhesives have not been used. Read labels carefully to avoid toxic materials. Avoid bedding made with acrylic, antimicrobial compounds (like triclosan), flame retardants, formaldehyde, heavy metals, memory foam, nylon, phenols, polyfluoroalkyl substances, plastics (phthalates), polyester, polyurethane foam, PVC, stain repellent, stain resistance treatments, synthetic foam, synthetic latex, vinyl, and VOCs. Even "plant-based memory foam" may only contain about 3 to 20 percent soy-based foam, and the rest may still be made from highly toxic polyurethane foam.

Toys

Children have less body mass than adults, so hazardous substances affect them disproportionately. Their bodies are developing rapidly, and even low-level exposures can interfere with growth. Items that children regularly come in close contact with, such as toys, are of particular concern.

Recent studies have revealed alarming levels of cadmium and lead in toys. Also of particular concern are plastics. Playing with plastic toys increases the level of flame-retardant residue in children's urine; toddlers are particularly susceptible to this contamination due to hand-to-mouth contact. Phthalates from plastic toys have been associated with developmental toxicity and endocrine disruption.

Choose toys made from natural materials such as linen, wool, cotton, and solid wood. Try beeswax crayons with natural plant pigment dyes. Removing all plastics at once may be a bit shocking for children, but you can do this in stages by removing toys your children no longer play with and phasing in nontoxic toys.

PLUSH TOYS. The stuffing in plush toys often tests high for PBDE. Both prenatal and childhood PBDE exposures are associated with poorer attention span, fine motor coordination, and cognition. Look for natural and organic stuffed toys instead.

BATH TOYS. When tested, more than half of flexible plastic bath toys that suck in water, like rubber duckies, had appreciable levels of fungi in them. Most of the bath toys tested also housed the bacteria *Pseudomonas aeruginosa*, which has been known to cause infections, especially in those with compromised immunity. Play it safe and keep plastic toys out of the bath.

TENTS AND SLEEPING BAGS. Tents, sleeping bags, and tentlike tunnel toys are made from plastics, which means phthalate exposure. When plastics heat up in sunlight or near a heater, they off-gas, and the weird odors this creates in the air is from chemicals. Organic cotton children's tents and teepees

are available as alternatives, and, of course, forts can be made "old-school" style with blankets and pillows.

COSTUMES. Packaged Halloween and dress-up costumes are made from plastic fabrics with plastic adornments, and the whole lot is surprisingly toxic, containing formaldehyde, heavy metals, parabens, and phthalates. Secondhand costumes that have already been through the wash many times have a lesser chemical burden. Making costumes from natural materials like paper and old fabric is safest.

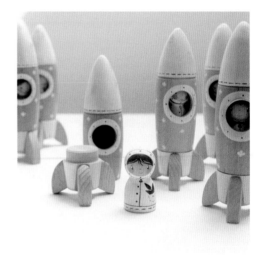

These handcrafted, nontoxic wooden toys are made to be passed down for generations.

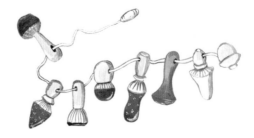

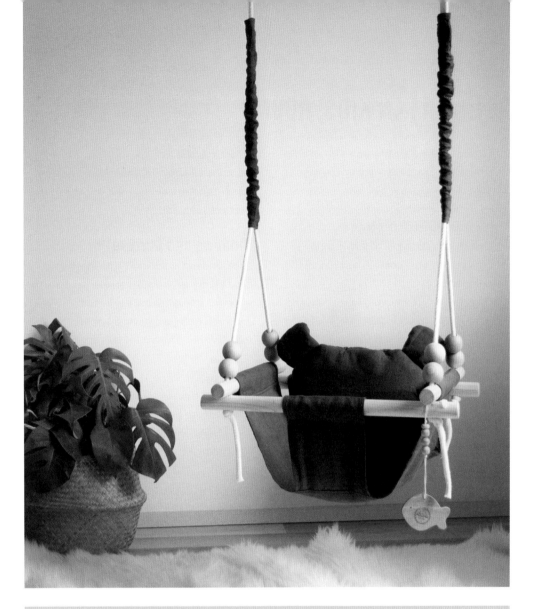

KID-FRIENDLY PLANTS

Add a few plants to your child's room to help clean the air. Plants absorb airborne toxins and produce clean oxygen, and they are more effective at removing solvents and flame retardants than many air filter systems. Some great air-purifying plants for kids' rooms are baby rubber plant, baby's tears, Boston fern, and spider plant.

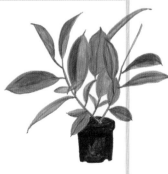

DETOX CLEAN KIDS' ROOMS

NOW THAT YOU HAVE REMOVED all the toxic items from your kids' rooms, you can focus on cleaning up the dust and residue from plastics, flame retardants, chemical cleaners, and germs. A thorough antibacterial wipe-down will remove all of this, creating a safe and healthy environment for children to play and rest.

Children's rooms are often full of gear and toys, and you will need to set aside plenty of time to clean each item in the room. It's much easier to clean a space properly when it's not full of unnecessary items, so continually remove items that your children no longer want or need.

Air

Open windows, and if you have a fan, turn it on while you clean.

Ceiling and Walls

Start high and work down. Remove light fixtures, clean out bugs and dust, and clean the glass. Then dust around the ceiling, corners, and walls. If the walls are painted (rather than papered), spray them with Tea Tree Wash (page 21) and wipe down with a clean dry cloth, replacing the cloth often to avoid spreading dust. Move dressers, toy bins, bookshelves, and bed frames so you can get behind them to wipe down the walls.

Floor and Carpet

Vacuum carpets and floors thoroughly. Vacuum rugs or shake them outside, wearing a mask to protect yourself from the dust. Vacuum behind and under all furniture. Spray a light misting of Tea Tree Wash on rugs and carpets to kill mites, bacteria, and fungi.

Windows and Mirrors

Clean windows and mirrors with Glass Spray (page 18). If there's visible mildew on or around windows, remove the mildew by spraying Tea Tree Wash and then wiping dry with a clean cloth. This helps inhibit future mildew growth.

Bedding

Clean bed frames and cribs by misting with Tea Tree Wash and wiping down all surfaces. Wash sheets, mattress pads, blankets, and pillows with hot water, Liquid Laundry Soap (page 19), and 10 drops of tea tree essential oil. Dry all bedding thoroughly; you can use wool dryer balls to reduce drying time.

Drawers

Remove all items from each dresser and table drawer and spray the interior with Tea Tree Wash. Wipe out and let dry thoroughly before replacing items.

Toys

Mist all toys with Tea Tree Wash and wipe dry using a clean cloth.

Books

Mist a cloth with Tea Tree Wash and use it to wipe down all book covers. If a book smells moldy, it will need to be thrown out to reduce further spread and growth of mold in the house. It is not possible to remove mildew from a book, and the spores can spread to other areas of the house unless they are removed.

Surfaces

Use Tea Tree Wash to mist all surfaces, including bookshelves, desktops, art tables, and cabinets. Wipe dry with a clean cloth.

GREAT JOB!

Take a few deep breaths and let your heart relax, knowing that you have created a truly clean and safe environment where your children can play and rest and grow.

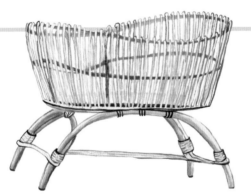

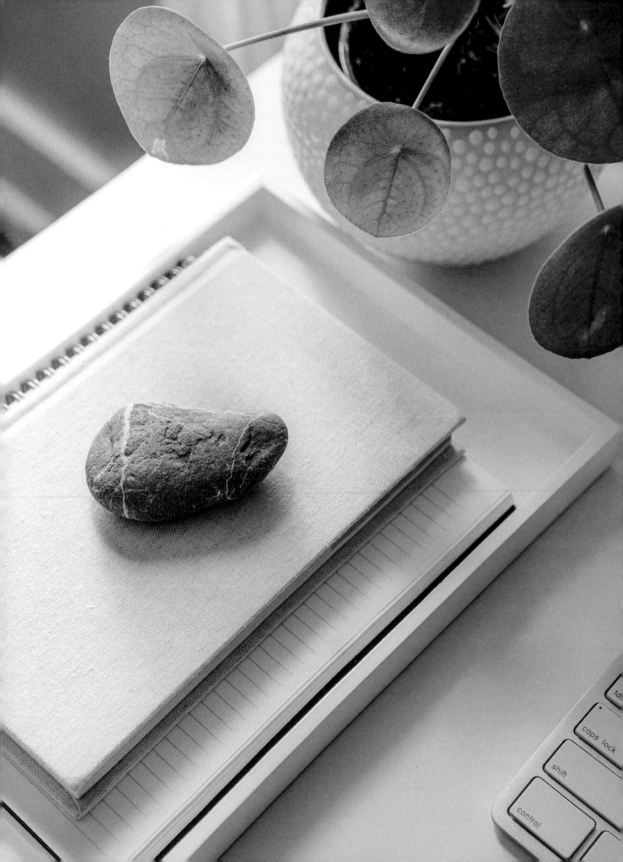

8

HOME OFFICE

Many of us are spending more time in a home office space, whether for work or for crafting and creating, so we need to carefully review the space for risks. It's important to ventilate the area often because there are many active sources of concern, including printers, electronics, and even art supplies.

HIDDEN TOXINS IN THE HOME OFFICE

UPHOLSTERED OFFICE CHAIRS, especially the less expensive ones sold at office supply stores, emit surprisingly high levels of flame retardants and VOCs from their polyurethane foam. If the room is not well ventilated, these gases and dust from foam and furniture can cause headaches, burning eyes, fatigue, and inflammation. Some other elusive concerns in the office include electromagnetic fields (EMFs) from computers and other electronics like modems, printers, scanners, cell phones, and cordless devices. Read Chapter 5 on living room furniture and adjust your home office furnishings accordingly.

Art Supplies

Home office spaces often do double duty for work and art. Art materials may contain heavy metals or solvents. Having anything poisonous in a house with children or pets is always a bit of a gamble due to accidental ingestion. My cat has walked right across a wet painting, leaving paw prints across my art table. Luckily, I was able to catch her and wash those paws before she licked them.

Any art supplies with a strong smell, like felt-tip pens, paint thinners, or glues, carry some risk due to VOCs and solvents. If you can detect an odor, know that you are inhaling the chemicals that create that odor into your lungs. Solvents should not be inhaled or allowed to touch the skin because they will be absorbed into the bloodstream. Even infrequent exposure to solvents can cause enough neurological damage to increase the risk for multiple sclerosis.

Oil-based paints are nontoxic when made from linseed, safflower, poppy, or walnut oil, but the pigments can still be toxic. Solvent-free gel medium and water-soluble oil paints are a few alternatives to the traditional oil paints and solvents.

Never wash toxic substances such as solvents down the sink or the toilet. These highly volatile chemicals must be disposed of properly at your local dump's toxic substance site. Consider switching to less toxic materials that require only water for cleanup, such as watercolor paints. Water-based paints do not require solvents for cleaning; plain tap water is sufficient. Acrylic paints are water based, but they do contain plastic. I personally prefer water-based, nontoxic, natural gouache paints for their rich colors, opacity, ability to layer color, and natural texture. And the pigments are intense, so only a tiny amount of paint is needed, which means I only need a small portable paint set.

Review your art supplies. Toss old materials that are no longer usable, make notes about items that need to be replaced, and then shop for nontoxic items.

TOXIC TEN

1. ART SUPPLIES
2. CARBON DIOXIDE
3. DUST
4. ELECTRONICS
5. EMFS
6. FURNITURE
7. PENS
8. PRINTERS
9. UPHOLSTERY
10. VOCS

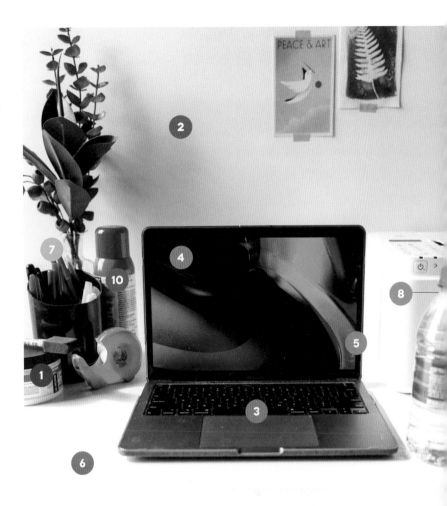

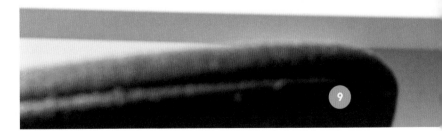

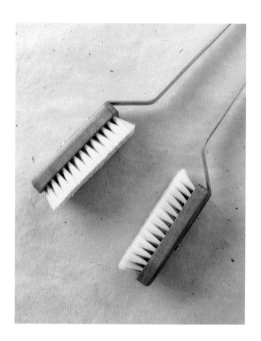

Carbon Dioxide (CO₂)

We produce CO_2 as we breathe, and this gas can build up in small, enclosed spaces, making us tired and foggy-brained. This situation is easily remedied with proper ventilation and houseplants. Open windows and doors and turn on fans to allow gases to escape and to bring in fresh air. Houseplants create an abundance of fresh oxygen and remove CO_2 and other air contaminants.

Use a soft brush to dust off plants. This keeps plants from looking dull; it also helps them take in light and improves their respiration so they can remove toxins from the air.

THE BEST HOUSEPLANTS TO REMOVE TOXINS

Houseplants are extraordinary air purifiers. The US National Aeronautics and Space Administration (NASA) studied houseplants to see how well they could detoxify the air for astronauts in space. They discovered that even plants that don't require a lot of light can remove VOC pollution from air, including even the most damaging compounds such as benzene, formaldehyde, and trichloroethylene (TCE). And these plants really do a thorough job; for example, one study showed that English ivy could remove 90 percent of the benzene from a room in just 24 hours.

Adding air-purifying plants to each room of your house will refresh the air and protect you from chemical exposures for many years. This is a beautiful example of how a simple, low-cost change can transform your life. The best plants for removing a wide range of air pollutants in your home include dragon tree, gerbera daisy, golden pothos, Janet Craig dracena, peace lily, snake plant, and warneckei.

Dust

Office dust is composed of particulates from plastic, brominated flame retardants (BFRs), paper, and human skin cells and hair. I spend a lot of time in my home office writing and painting, so when I started having frequent headaches, it was the first place I looked for potential causes. The deeper I looked, the more I found. The room had several areas that I couldn't vacuum easily due to heavy furniture and old wall-to-wall carpet that never stained no matter how many times my cat barfed on it. This was a huge clue that the carpet was treated with PFOAs. Once I moved the drawers, bookshelves, and two desks, I could see that cat hair and an amazing amount of dust had been trapped there for years. This is embarrassing to admit, but the total amount of yuck that I vacuumed up filled my vacuum canister. I am currently in the process of replacing the old carpet in my house with wood floors, one area at a time to spread out the cost. I also added casters to the drawer units to make them easy to move for cleaning. My headaches and my sinus issues always improve after removing dust.

Electronics

Most of us use laptops, smartphones, and other electronics all day. This puts them on the Toxic Ten list simply because longer exposure will have a greater effect on your health. EMFs aside, electronic devices that have plastic parts, like monitors and casings, contain BFRs. As the plastic heats up, it releases tiny particles, which gather in the dust that circulates around the room. Cleaning dust from electronics in the

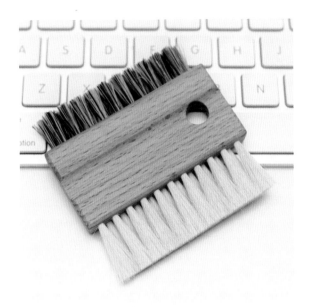

Keyboard brushes work well to sweep away crumbs and dust. Cans of aerosol spray are not needed; they contain propellants and chemicals that have negative impacts on the environment.

office seems like a no-brainer, but we tend to forget about it because it can be hard to see and accumulates in hard-to-reach places.

Electromagnetic Fields (EMFs)

EMFs arise from radio waves, television signals, microwaves, cordless telephones, cell phone towers, two-way radios, radar, Bluetooth devices, computers, tablets, cell phones, modems, and routers. Exposure to EMFs has been linked to headaches, anxiety, and even tumor growth. It's also thought to cause fetal development damage, which has spurred many countries to warn pregnant women to wear a shield around their bellies when using personal electronic devices.

Electronic technology has developed rapidly and is now ubiquitous, so at this time we may not be able to completely avoid EMFs, but we can reduce our exposure. For example, we can tap into the internet through a fiber-optic connection, which uses light rather than electricity. We can use a cable to connect a computer to a modem, rather than using Wi-Fi. We can turn off the modem and all other electronics at night to shut down all exposure for those hours while we sleep. We can create distance between our bodies and our devices by using the speaker function on our cell phones, rather than holding them to our ears, and carrying them in a purse or backpack rather than keeping them close to our bodies. And we can use a desktop computer rather than a laptop, so our bodies are physically distanced by those extra inches of space.

Furniture

Office desks, cabinets, and bookshelves are often made from composite materials that contain wood particles, plastics, and glues. Upholstered furniture like cushy desk chairs, sofas, and ottomans usually contain polyurethane foam. These materials all create toxic dust.

If you already have composite-material furniture and you suspect that you're reacting to it, try ventilating the room with fans or by opening windows and doors to reduce your exposure. If you are immune compromised or chemically sensitive, you may need to switch out the offending items and replace them with more inert (metal or wood) furniture.

If you want to replace items, look for solid wood, metal, bamboo, upcycled items from thrift stores, hand-me-downs, or antiques.

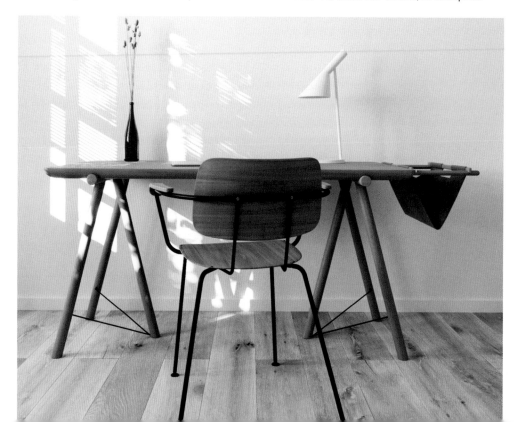

Pens

Highlighters and markers contain toxic chemicals like xylene, which is why we can get dizzy from sniffing them. Aromas of potent chemical scents are clues that we are breathing in something bad. If we didn't have that warning sign, it would be much harder to remember that something as seemingly innocent as art or office supplies could be a source of risk. Emissions from felt-tip markers and white-board markers are neurotoxic and can trigger behavioral abnormalities such as altered posture and gait, tremors, falling, and hyperactivity due to their alcohols, acetates, and ketones. Washable and odorless markers are safer as they do not contain VOCs.

Printers

Copiers, scanners, and printers are often wireless, which means they are sending out electrical signals to other devices, such as your laptop. I used an EMF meter and found that my inkjet printer was putting out high-level EMFs. After that, I started to turn off the printer when I wasn't using it. Then I switched to a laser printer that has a button to enable Wi-Fi so I can easily turn that function off, which cuts the EMFs to almost nothing.

Printers also emit solvents and VOCs from the ink cartridges. Houseplants, which absorb airborne solvents and VOCs, will help keep the air in the office clean (see the list on page 128). Ventilate the room to release trapped airborne chemicals and printer paper dust.

Upholstery

As discussed in the living room chapter (see page 93), furniture that has cushioning, like those big comfortable desk chairs, contains polyurethane foam that is likely treated with flame-retardant chemicals that off-gas and shed toxic foam particles that become part of the house dust. If the foam-filled furniture and fabric-covered items in your office are treated with stain-resistant coatings, they carry the additional risk of PFAS that emit VOCs into the room for years.

Solid wood and metal chairs with a wool seat cushion are nontoxic options.

VOCs

Collectively, the level of VOCs from furniture, pens, printers, and upholstery can be significant in our home offices, especially if fragrances, synthetic carpets and rugs, sofas, candles, or incense are also in this space. Our office spaces are typically small and often lack cross-ventilation because we close the doors for quiet and privacy as we work. Consider the concentration of fragrances and airborne toxins in your office and start to detoxify this room with ventilation. Crack open windows and turn on a fan, and reduce the chemical load by removing and replacing items to eliminate the source.

DETOX CLEAN THE HOME OFFICE

ANY ROOM where we spend a lot of time will have a high moisture level from our body heat and breath. Heat and moisture encourage mold growth, so keep an eye out for mold in hidden areas, around cords, behind desks, on windowsills, and near floorboards. Office items create a lot of toxic particles, so focus on tracking down all that dust.

Air

Ventilate the room by opening windows and doors to allow fumes to escape and reduce your exposure to toxic particulates in the air. If you don't have at least two openings to create cross-ventilation, use fans to help move the air. If you don't have a window in the room, be sure to use an air purifier. If you have composite-material furniture and you suspect that you're reacting to it, ventilate the room for an hour before you start cleaning. Dust will be stirred up as you clean, and ventilating reduces your exposure while you are cleaning.

Ceiling and Walls

Start high and work down. Remove light fixtures, clean out bugs and dust, and clean the glass. Then dust around the ceiling, corners, and walls. If the walls are painted (rather than papered), spray them with Tea Tree Wash (page 21) and wipe down with a clean dry cloth, replacing the cloth often to avoid spreading dust. Move desks, shelves, cabinets, sofas, and other furniture as needed to wipe down the walls behind them.

Floors and Carpet

Start by vacuuming nooks and crannies with an attachment, then vacuum the floors and carpets. A thorough vacuuming removes most of the dust from a room, and this one step alone can reduce asthma symptoms and burning eyes. Rooms with heavy furniture, such as desks and shelves, often get only a cursory vacuuming and dust bunnies collect in the spaces between furniture and walls. Some of this material will make its way out into the room and the air you breathe, so it's worth the effort to reach the hidden pockets and remove as much dust as possible.

Surfaces

Mist all hard surfaces with Tea Tree Wash, including desktops, lamp bases, and shelving. Clean all items, such as vases, sculpture, and trays. This will remove dust and also eliminate bacteria, viruses, and mold.

Drawers

Remove all items from each drawer and spray the interiors with Tea Tree Wash. Wipe out and let dry thoroughly before replacing items.

Windows and Mirrors

Clean windows and mirrors with Glass Spray (page 18). If there's visible mildew on or around windows, remove the mildew by spraying Tea Tree Wash and then wiping dry with a clean cloth. This removes the mold and helps inhibit future mildew growth.

Window Coverings

Wash the office curtains regularly. If you have pets or smokers in the house, the curtains will likely need a monthly trip to the washing machine. If you locate mold anywhere in the room, wash the curtains with hot water, laundry soap, and 10 drops of tea tree essential oil. Dry the curtains thoroughly before rehanging them, as damp fabrics become a breeding ground for microbial growth.

Blinds and shutters gather dust and mold. Vacuum with a brush attachment to remove dust. Mist every surface with Tea Tree Wash and wipe down with dry cloths to remove all particles of dust, microbes, and other toxins.

TAKE A DEEP BREATH

This is where you work and create. Let your mind relax, knowing that this space is now safe, fresh, and clean. Enjoy.

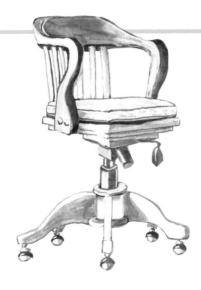

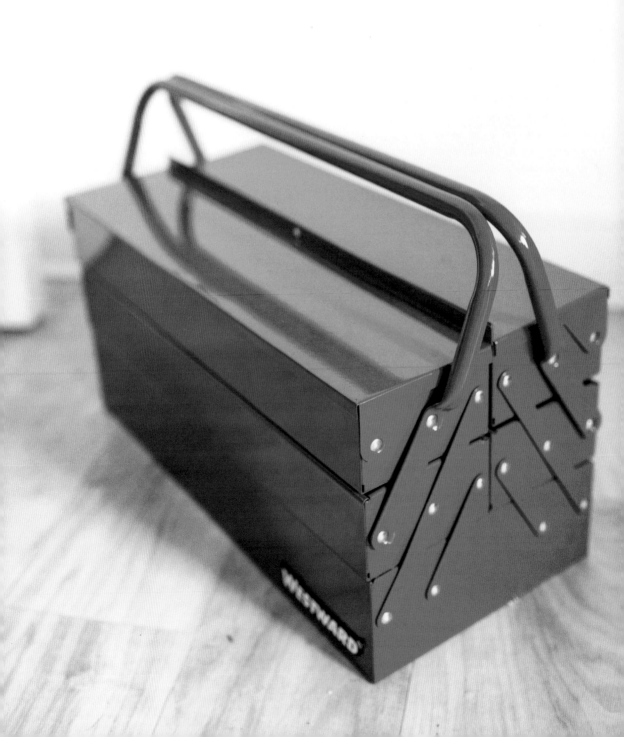

9
GARAGE AND BASEMENT

We sure do like to hang on to stuff, as evidenced by the number of storage units we fill with the things we don't really need anymore. Hopefully, you can shake loose some attachments and free yourself from the burden of *stuff*. Fewer items means a healthier home with less dust and fewer chemicals, and it will be easier to clean properly.

HIDDEN TOXINS IN THE GARAGE AND BASEMENT

OUR GARAGES AND BASEMENTS can become deadly storage areas, housing solvents linked to neurological disorders, pest poisons that cause cancer and kill pets, and fumes that affect our ability to use oxygen properly. Over time, products for home improvement, repairs, and auto care pile up and may stay on shelves for years. I have found products in my clients' homes that were so old they contained ingredients that had been banned for decades. Going through each of them and determining what to eliminate is a satisfying job. Be sure to dispose of each item in a way that is safe for the environment. This will also clear space for your new, less toxic gear.

Some of the top concerns in these spaces, like radon and carbon monoxide, may require lab tests to identify levels. Lab test recommendations are listed in the Resources section on page 164.

Antifreeze

Most formulations of this helpful but potentially deadly solution contain ethylene glycol as their main ingredient. This chemical compound is used to make not only antifreeze (aka engine coolant) but also polyester fibers, and it is highly toxic to humans and animals. Ingestion causes irreversible kidney damage in pets. The sweet smell of ethylene glycol attracts animals, but it is deadly if ingested even in small amounts. As little as half a teaspoon of antifreeze can kill a cat, and eight ounces can kill a 75-pound dog. Spilled or leaked antifreeze washes into rivers and lakes, harming fish and other wildlife.

Keep an eye out for any small green puddles in the garage or on the pavement where cars are parked. Leaks from engine coolant systems are not common, but small spills may occur when you're topping off the car's coolant reservoir. Opt instead for antifreeze formulations made with propylene glycol, which are less toxic and just as effective as those made with ethylene glycol, though a little more expensive.

Carbon Monoxide

Carbon monoxide (CO) gas is created as a result of combustion of coal, natural gas, and oil. This airborne toxin comes from many sources in the home and creates a health risk. According to the Environmental Protection Agency, symptoms of CO exposure include fatigue, chest pain, impaired vision, incoordination, dizziness, nausea, confusion, and headaches. Symptoms may also include mood changes, cognitive and personality changes, incontinence, dementia, and psychosis. High levels of exposure can even be fatal.

Dangerous levels of CO can be produced by any fuel-burning appliance, including gas furnaces, gas stoves, gas dryers, gas water heaters, and gas fireplaces. When these appliances have cracks, they leak gas into the home's air. Signs of a leak include heavy condensation or sooty stains near appliances or an exhaust odor. One visual sign of incomplete combustion in a furnace is a yellow burner flame instead of a clear blue flame. However, the safest way to tell if you have a CO leak is by installing carbon monoxide detectors in your home.

TOXIC TEN

1. ANTIFREEZE
2. CARBON MONOXIDE
3. MILDEW
4. PAINT
5. RADON
6. RODENTICIDES
7. RUST REMOVER
8. SOLVENTS
9. TIRES
10. WINDSHIELD WIPER FLUID

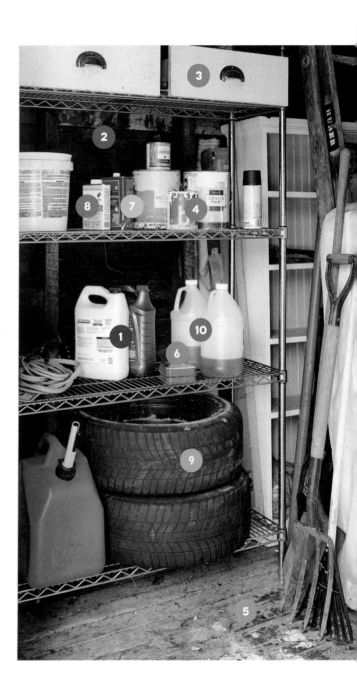

BEWARE CARBON MONOXIDE

I saw the dangers of CO firsthand when a client, a young woman, called me to report that she was feeling extremely ill, but her doctor couldn't make sense of her symptoms. She didn't have a fever, yet she was nauseous and pale, couldn't think clearly, felt dizzy, and was so weak she couldn't go to work. This athletic woman was too weak to take her dog out for walks. We brought in a contractor to investigate her home, and he immediately identified an old furnace that was leaking carbon monoxide into her living quarters. Fortunately, her cabin had large gaps around the door and window frames, which had allowed enough airflow that she was not seriously harmed. She replaced the furnace, and her symptoms cleared up immediately.

Portable generators used during power outages are notorious for causing carbon monoxide poisoning. The exhaust from a generator is a potent source of CO, and if the exhaust is forced or trapped inside a home, it may cause illness or death. Only run a generator outside and make sure it is at least 20 feet from any window or door. Keep an extension cord that is at least 20 feet long stored with the generator so that you will be ready to power your appliances from an appropriate distance in an emergency.

Cars are also a common source of CO in homes. When garages are attached to homes, they become a significant source of CO from automobile exhaust that drifts into living spaces. CO and other combustion pollutants can be drawn into the home through an open door that leads directly from the garage and into the home, but they can also seep in through gaps around doors, ductwork, and other openings. These leaks can be hard to find and are tough to seal. If you have an attached garage, protect your household by installing a CO detector in your home and consider parking your car in the driveway instead of the garage to reduce the risk of CO exposure.

Mildew

Basements and garages are often poorly lit, so water leaks may go unnoticed. Stagnant water collects mold spores that can grow into full-fledged mildew that can develop quickly on porous surfaces like drywall, wood, and concrete. Remediate growth by first removing the water and drying the area with fans and open windows. If you can smell mildew, you may need to set up an air purifier to remove spores. To keep air dry, consider a reusable silica gel desiccant. Once the moisture is under control, mist the area with diluted tea tree essential oil: 1 part tea tree essential oil to 1 part water. This will help kill the remaining spores and prevent regrowth. Check the area weekly to make sure it remains dry and mold-free. Use tea tree essential oil as necessary to stop any new growth.

Paint

Paints contain solvents that release volatile organic compounds (VOCs) while the paint is wet and even once it is dry. Look for low-VOC and zero-VOC paint, ventilate while applying it, and wear a mask when spray painting and sanding. Be aware of paint removal products, as their solvents are highly toxic. Lacquer thinner, commonly used for removing household paints, is known to contain a mixture of various hydrocarbons and naphtha. Children are particularly susceptible, and solvents and paint thinners have compounds known to increase the risk of childhood leukemia.

Radon

Radon is the principal cause of lung cancer in nonsmokers and the second most common cause in smokers. In outdoor air, radon is diluted and is not a health concern, but as it leaks into houses, the gas accumulates, reaching high concentrations, and becomes a health hazard. Use a radon home lab test kit, especially in the basement where radon can become trapped and concentrated.

Rodenticides

Walk down the aisle of the hardware store where products are sold to kill mice, rats,

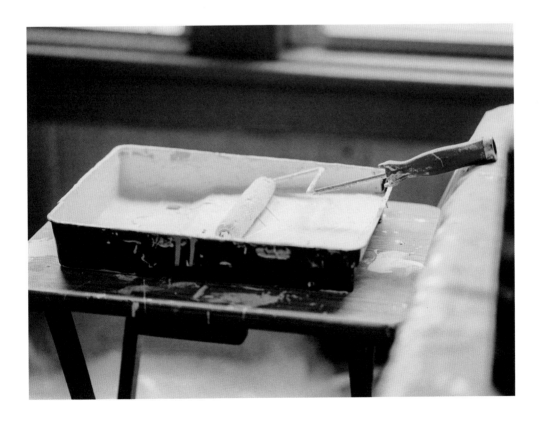

moles, and gophers, and you will be able to smell the poison. These chemicals cause horrific suffering to wild animals, create a toxic food chain when dogs, cats, foxes, owls, eagles, or other predators eat the poisoned animals, and add toxicity to the soil, also inadvertently poisoning bees.

There's no need for rodenticides. Small animals are highly sensitive to strong smells and are easily deterred by essential oils. Mist eucalyptus, lavender, or tea tree essential oil around the vents, windows, and doors. Reapply the essential oils about once a month. This is an effective, nontoxic, and inexpensive strategy for repelling small animals.

Rust Remover

Rust is created by oxidation. It's not only unsightly but also weakens and corrodes metals. If rust is removed before it does damage, you might save a bicycle or a wheelbarrow. But rust removal products are bad news because they contain caustic ingredients including hydrochloric acid and sulfuric acid. Steel wool, sandpaper, and Tub Scrub (page 21) are all abrasives that work well for removing a layer of rust. If that doesn't do the trick, try white vinegar. Its acetic acid will dissolve rust.

Solvents

A solvent is a substance that dissolves another substance. We find them in many everyday products, including nail polish remover, printer ink, cleaning products, art supplies, rust remover, and paint thinners.

Solvents vaporize easily and stay in the air for months. Immediate symptoms of toxic exposure to solvents include feeling light-headed, dizzy spells, nausea, and vomiting, and long-term exposure can lead to neurological problems and potentially the development of neurological diseases, including multiple sclerosis. So if you smell solvents, such as turpentine, in your garage, hunt down the source and remove it.

Avoid products that contain solvents by reading labels and being on the lookout for benzene (found in paint, glues, detergents), perfluorooctane (in ski wax and water-resistant sprays for sportswear), toluene (in nail polish remover), turpentine (a paint thinner), and xylene (in paint and varnish). Use nontoxic alternatives, such as water-based glues, natural cleaning supplies, plant-based wax or beeswax, and water-based paint, which requires only water for cleanup.

Tires

Decades of research have gone into finding the cause of Coho salmon deaths in the rivers and streams around Puget Sound. A chemical compound from car tires, 6PPD-quinone, has been contaminating streams and killing the salmon before they could spawn.

When we drive, the friction of tires on the road leaves behind particulates of the tire materials. Runoff from roads carries particulates directly into waterways. At the same time, 60 million tires are degrading in landfills in the United States, releasing micro- and nanoplastics into our environment.

I wondered what specific chemicals tires emit, so I ordered a lab test kit and took it to my local tire center to find out. The test required a 24-hour collection of air. Keep in mind this was only an air sample and not even actual tire material being tested. The results showed 76 toxic compounds, including high levels of benzene, hexane, and xylene. These chemicals are polluting our environment, and we breathe them every time we drive our cars. Tires stored in enclosed spaces like a garage or basement release these same pollutants. Consider storing your snow tires in an open-air carport or in mini storage to reduce exposure.

Biking, walking, and riding public transportation are short-term solutions. Hopefully, with advances in mushroom-based plastic alternatives, hemp bioplastics, and other plant-based materials, we will soon have better options.

Windshield Wiper Fluid

Have you ever wondered what keeps windshield wiper fluid from freezing? It's the same chemical used in car radiators to keep water from freezing: ethylene glycol or propylene glycol. The skull-and-crossbones on the packaging lets us know that ethylene glycol is poisonous.

Propylene glycol is much less toxic than ethylene glycol, but it still comes in a plastic jug, so I wondered about a DIY solution. I tested a small amount of vinegar in water, and it worked like a charm as windshield wiper fluid. Water alone will work to clean off dust, and vinegar helps if lots of bugs or sap won't rinse off with water. However, during cold months when the temperature drops below freezing, propylene glycol is necessary to keep your wiper fluid from freezing.

• ● •

WINDSHIELD WIPER FLUID

Keep in mind this is only for use in warmer months when temperatures are above freezing.

1 part white vinegar
3 parts water

Combine the vinegar and water and fill your car's windshield wiper fluid reservoir with this solution.

DETOX CLEAN THE GARAGE AND BASEMENT

GARAGES AND BASEMENTS can be wastelands for unused items, cleaning products, and yard and automotive products, as well as the dust and grime from these items. As you remove items, you may uncover hidden messes that need attention. A deep clean will remediate these and allow you to organize the space and gain easy access to the items you need.

Air

Open windows and doors and turn on a fan to let dust escape as you clean.

Ceiling and Walls

Start high and work down. Remove light fixtures, clean out bugs and dust, and clean the glass. Then dust around the ceiling, corners, and walls. If the walls are painted (rather than papered), spray them with Tea Tree Wash (page 21) and wipe down with a clean dry cloth, replacing the cloth often to avoid spreading dust. Move items like shelves, boxes, and tool chests as needed so you can clean behind them.

Floor

Sweep or vacuum the floor, paying special attention to the corners, and hunt down any dust and cobwebs that have collected.

There may be oil spots from the car, solvents that have leaked from cans, or cleaning products that have dropped onto surfaces or floors. Look for them. If you can smell any chemical, it's there and must be removed. Sprinkle baking soda on oily or liquid spills to soak them up; you can even leave a thick coat of baking soda on the spill overnight, then sweep it up the next day. Use Tub Scrub as an abrasive to remove spills, and if necessary, use a small amount of a natural citrus-based solvent to remove light oil stains. Follow the directions on the bottle and vent the area well as you use the natural solvent.

Let the space air out completely and make sure all surfaces are dry before putting items back in their place. When you replace bottles on shelves, make sure they are sitting flat to avoid spills. If you have windows in your garage or basement, consider hanging a few spider plants to help keep the air fresh and clean.

NICE GOING!

This is a big job for most folks, so give yourself a high five. Rest assured that you can breathe deeply and count on these workhorse spaces to be areas where you will feel good when you spend time in them.

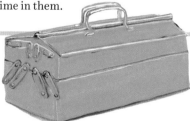

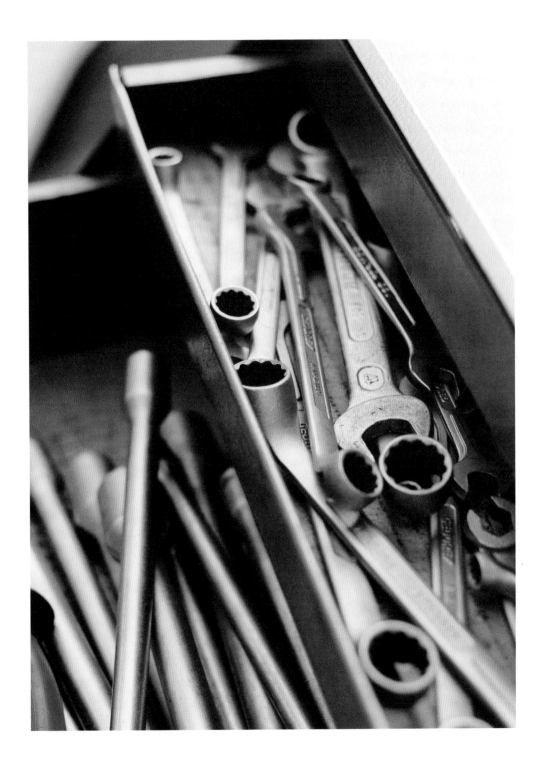

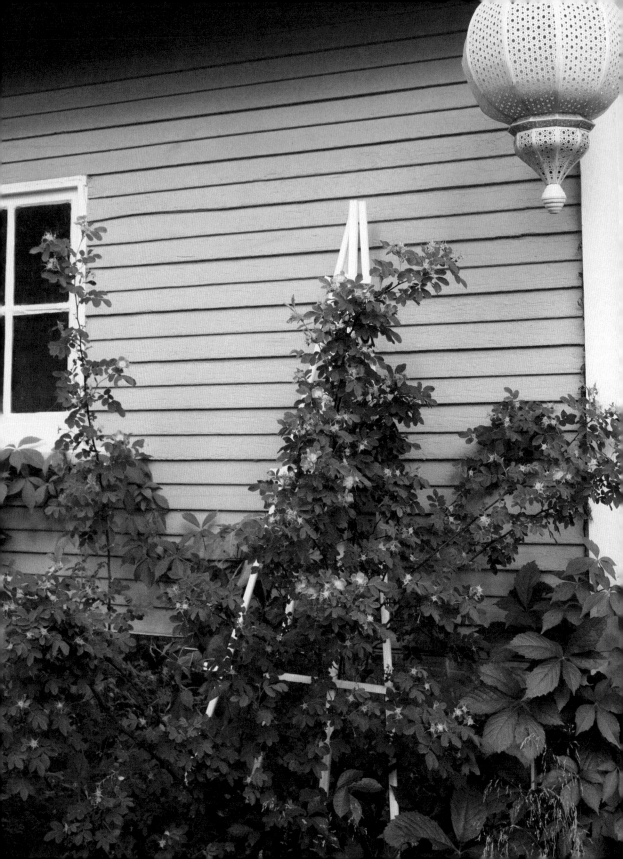

10
YARD AND GARDEN

It's easy to forget about toxic exposures when we're outside. We might be paying more attention to our gardens, watching kids play on the swing set, reading a book and relaxing on the deck, or grilling a good meal. Most of us are blissfully unaware of warning signs in our own yards, such as chemical smells, smoke, or drifting chemicals from surrounding areas.

HIDDEN TOXINS IN THE YARD AND GARDEN

THE REASSURING ASPECT of making changes outside the house is that we can resolve common problems and clean up exposures with a few broad strokes to protect ourselves, our families, our pets, and the wildlife in our neighborhoods.

But our outdoor environment stretches beyond our yards. Consider that pesticides and herbicides from neighbors a mile away can affect our risk of cancer and affect fetal development. If you know your neighbors, you might consider sharing what you've learned to expand the safe zone around your home out into the neighborhood. A couple of ways to start the conversation are to share this book, share research, and offer alternatives to those who are open to making change but aren't aware of their options. In my little village of Port Townsend, Washington, many of my neighbors post "Pesticide-Free Zone" signs to let others know they do not use chemicals in their yards. It catches on.

Bug Repellent

Insects can be annoying, especially in large numbers. Some, such as mosquitos, fleas, and ticks, can also be worrisome because they transmit pathogens like parasites and bacteria, including *Bartonella* bacteria and babesiosis. Enormous efforts have been taken to develop effective repellents against arthropods, and it's no wonder we jumped at an insecticide like N,N-diethyl-meta-toluamide (DEET). Like many so-called magic bullets brought to us by chemical corporations, though, DEET has a downside. It poses vast environmental and health risks and is now known to be toxic, particularly for infants and pregnant women.

Fortunately, we have good nontoxic alternatives to use as bug repellents. Coconut oil is highly effective, widely available, and inexpensive. Coconut fatty acids are active against a broad array of blood-sucking arthropods, including biting flies, ticks, bedbugs, and mosquitoes. It repels biting flies and bedbugs for two weeks after application, and ticks for one week. This natural oil repels with a stronger and longer-lasting residual activity than that of DEET. Researchers found that even diluted coconut fatty acids protect pastured cattle from biting flies for up to 96 hours in the hot summer, which is the longest protection provided by a natural repellent product studied to date.

Plant-based repellents have been tested in many trials, and numerous essential oils have been found effective in repelling bugs, including citronella, pine, and peppermint, which provided complete protection against mosquitoes for over 9 hours.

TOXIC TEN

1. **BUG REPELLENT**
2. **CHEMICAL FERTILIZERS**
3. **FIRE PIT**
4. **GARDEN HOSE**
5. **PESTICIDES**
6. **GAS GRILLS**
7. **HERBICIDES**
8. **PLASTIC TOYS**
9. **PLAY SETS**
10. **TREATED WOOD**

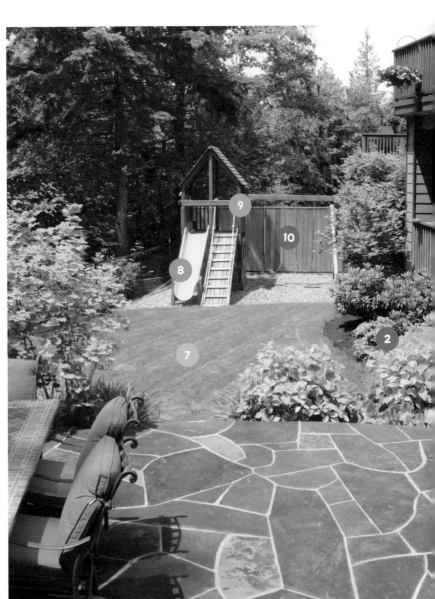

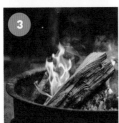

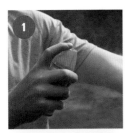

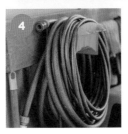

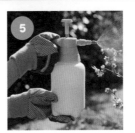

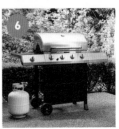

• ● •

ESSENTIAL OIL BUG SPRAY

Essential oils are concentrated and should be diluted with water, especially when used around children. Some oils are more irritating for children than others; eucalyptus and rosemary are not recommended for children under the age of 10.

1 ounce water

1–2 drops of an essential oil

Basil	Eucalyptus	Peppermint
Cedar	Jasmine	Pine
Chamomile	Juniper	Rosemary
Cinnamon	Lavender	Sandalwood
Citronella	Lemongrass	Tea tree
Clove	Mint	

Combine the water and essential oil in a small spray bottle. Shake well and mist on skin as needed to repel bugs.

Chemical Fertilizers

Many chemical fertilizers are poisonous to humans, pets, and wildlife, especially those containing organophosphates. Instead use compost as a natural and nutrient-rich fertilizer, and add organic mycorrhizal inoculant root enhancer to boost plant growth.

Fire Pit

Sitting around a fire warming my toes after skiing is a fond memory for me. In retrospect, I have to admit that it always made me cough, my eyes burned, and I felt hungover after those smoky festivities. Years later, I began to understand the connection. Smoke from any source, whether forest fire, fire pit, grill, or bonfire, produces polycyclic aromatic hydrocarbons (PAHs), which are complex environmental toxicants generated during the burning of organic materials (coal, oil, gas, and wood). Many PAHs can damage DNA, increase cancer risk, and trigger an immune response. PAHs are highly lipid soluble, which means that they are absorbed into the blood easily and stored in body fat. Even a short exposure is enough to trigger inflammatory responses for many people, such as migraines, muscle pain, and foggy brain. So if you are burning things outside, be sure to stay out of the smoke and only burn clean organic material, such as firewood and branches, which produces the least amount of smoke. Do not burn plastics, painted wood, plywood, and treated wood.

As a health care practitioner, I advise my clients who are reactive to PAHs to take antioxidants as soon as they are aware of the exposure to help the body excrete the PAHs and reduce the potential for inflammation. Antioxidants are found in fruits and vegetables, including blueberries, leafy greens, and citrus, or supplements such as quercetin, vitamin C, or N-acetylcysteine (NAC).

Garden Hose

Hoses are so much more toxic than I ever would have dreamed. If only I had known this when I was a kid and drank right out of the hose in my backyard!

The first clue that a hose is contaminated will likely come from your nose. Hose water has a distinctive chemical smell, and in fact, the average garden hose delivers a cocktail of toxins. In 2016 the Ecology Center in Ann Arbor, Michigan, tested 32 new garden hoses from major retailers and found that many PVC hoses contain high levels of bromine (indicating BFRs), lead, antimony, tin, and phthalates. A majority of the hoses had chemical levels deemed "high concern."

Thirty percent of the hoses tested contained more than 100 ppm lead, which is the threshold set by the US Consumer Product Safety Commission (CPSC) standard for lead in children's products. Water samples from the hoses had lead levels 18 times higher than the federal drinking water standard. This is concerning because lead causes neurological and kidney damage, high blood pressure, disrupted blood cell production, and reproductive problems. In addition, di(2-ethylhexyl) phthalate (DEHP) was found at a level four times higher, and bisphenol A (BPA) at a level 20 times higher, than federal drinking water standards.

The upside to this research was the discovery that polyurethane hoses labeled "drinking water safe" contained no chemicals of concern. When you're shopping for a new hose, look for a non-PVC hose made of polyurethane and labeled "drinking water safe." Paying more for a quality natural rubber hose will protect children, wildlife, garden plants, and the garden food we eat. It also will last much longer than the cheaper, thinner plastic hoses that kink and break.

Gas Grills

We've known for some time that propane emits high levels of PAHs, which create free radicals in our bodies when we breathe propane fumes. Gas grills also create carbon monoxide, which may not be a problem outdoors, but when grills are used in enclosed areas such as shacks, garages, or tents, or too close to a building, the gas can build up and be lethal. Another concern when grilling are the carcinogens that form when food is cooked with very high heat. The black material that forms when meat is charred has been linked to cancer. Keep a close eye on food as you are grilling so you can remove it before it burns and you will be able to avoid charring.

Herbicides

No one should use synthetic chemicals made to kill plants. They are too dangerous, even in small amounts. They damage all life on the planet. Glyphosate is the most widely used broad-spectrum systemic herbicide in the world. The World Health Organization (WHO) recently put out a warning for glyphosate-based weed killers, stating that they increase the risk of several common cancers by more than 40 percent. Even with the warning label, many people continue to apply these carcinogenic killers with little sense of the danger.

Numerous serious health issues have been proven to be linked to exposure to glyphosate-based herbicides, including and especially Roundup. Glyphosate can block the vitamin A pathways that are crucial for normal fetal development. The risk of brain cancer increases with exposure. Cancer rates are much higher in geographic areas where Roundup is used. A disruption of the biosynthesis of amino acids is linked to heart disease. Even very low doses of Roundup show a disruption of liver cell function. Glyphosate can impact sperm production and decrease testosterone.

NATURAL ALTERNATIVES TO HERBICIDES. Reducing the use of chemicals in our lives requires a new way of thinking, not simply finding replacement products that are less dangerous. For example, we can plant native plants that have a natural resistance to pests rather than buy plants that need pest management. Another idea: I use salt to kill the weeds in my gravel driveway. It's inexpensive and safe, takes very little to be effective, and the deer in my neighborhood love to come by for a little lick of salt after I sprinkle it on the gravel.

Pesticides

Synthetic chemicals developed to kill pests are highly poisonous to all living things and to the environment. We are exposed to these chemicals through inhaling sprayed dust, drift, skin contact, and eating foods that have been sprayed or grown in pesticide-treated soil. They are absorbed into the bloodstream easily and stored in body fat.

Pesticides play a significant role in some of our most devastating epidemics, including diabetes, cancer, and autism. First, pesticides contain heavy metals like arsenic, barium, lead, and a toxic form of zinc, which are neurotoxins. Sadly, many public areas, urban soil, schoolyards, and residential parks have been found to have high levels of heavy metals due to pesticide use.

Organochlorine pesticides (OCPs) and polycyclic aromatic hydrocarbons (PAHs) are some of the most concerning environmental pollutants because they are highly toxic and they bioacumulate. Exposure to them is linked to diseases of the skin, liver, and immune system, as well as asthma, migraines, inflammation, and cancer. They cause cancer because they are genotoxic and mutagenic. One of the most critical issues with pesticides is that they are persistent organic pollutants, meaning that they stick around for a long time. Many countries are aware of these issues and are actively fighting to ban pesticides.

HEALTHY PEST MANAGEMENT. If pests like fleas, mites, or ants have come into your house, essential oils can be used in diluted form and misted on floors, counters, and carpets. In the case of a flea or mite infestation, food-grade diatomaceous earth can be sprinkled on carpets; it works as a desiccant on larva to stop the breeding cycle. Sprinkle a light layer on every inch of carpet and leave it for a few hours. Then vacuum it up.

Food particles and residues attract a lot of hungry critters, such as ants and mice. If you find that they're congregating in a particular spot in your home, vacuum it well, then mist it with Tea Tree Wash (page 21) and wipe the area clean to remove all traces of food.

If you have a problem with insects in your yard, play detective and try to find the breeding ground. Mosquitoes, for example, hatch in standing water, so search out pools of water, buckets, or any item that holds standing water and eliminate it.

In gardens, healthy soil with high levels of microbes is like magic for improving the health of plants and managing pests. Biochar and beneficial mycorrhizae improve the health of plants in your garden so that they can fight pests naturally. Essential oils work well to deter critters like mice and rabbits. A spray of diluted Dr. Bronner's Sal Suds will often do the trick with aphids, caterpillars, crickets, and flies; mix 1 tablespoon Sal Suds with 1 cup water and spray on the leaves

of plants. This will desiccate insects' soft bodies and kill them without damaging the plant. Diatomaceous earth will eradicate fleas and mites.

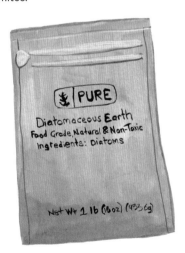

Diatomaceous earth is simply algae shells from the ocean. Under a microscope, diatoms are gorgeous tiny glass houses in a million different forms. These silica shells are powdered and sprinkled into soil to kill slugs, snails, and other small garden pests.

Plastic Toys

When I was young, I loved the bright colors of the toys advertised on Saturday-morning television. They were all made of plastic, so I thought all toys were plastic. Years later, while I was studying natural health sciences at Bastyr University, I was a nanny for a family whose children played with toys made of natural materials like wood, cotton, and wool. This was a huge awakening for me. Their philosophy was that toys made of natural materials help kids feel a connection to the natural world. They learn that wool comes from sheep and is made into yarn to be made into dolls, and that wood comes from trees and is carved into toys. They learn that when toys get old or broken, they can be repaired, or they can be composted because they are biodegradable. I was thrilled by this discovery. It was so far removed from what I had learned as a kid, and this new awareness changed the way I thought about the things I purchased.

So many of the outdoor toys sold for kids today are made of plastic. These toys are short lived and breakable, which means they end up in landfills. They also contain dangerous levels of phthalates and other chemicals of concern. If you have an outdoor pool, the inflatable pool toys and swimming devices like armbands, foam kickboards, and noodles can leak hazardous organic solvents. Those bitter odors you smell on plastic are the actual molecules of toxic compounds entering your nose. The pools themselves, if they are aboveground, are usually made of phthalates and polyvinyl chloride (PVC), which contain acutely toxic chemicals.

Play Sets

Play sets and climbing structures are typically made of wood, metal, or plastic. The wood sets are often built with pressure-treated wood, which contains heavy metals, and the plastic sets contain phthalates. Concern about children's exposure to arsenic from wood treated with chromated copper arsenate (CCA) led to a withdrawal of its approval for residential use in 2004. However, due to its effectiveness as an anti-rot treatment, millions of American homes still have CCA wood decks on which children play. Playgrounds built prior to 2004 with pressure-treated wood contain CCA and release arsenic into the soil. Surface soil near and underneath the structures has contained dangerously high levels of arsenic for decades. As the structures age, they release more arsenic into the soil where children play.

There are alternatives. Look for products from members of the US Green Building Council, and for play structures that use long-lasting Forest Stewardship Council–certified wood, recycled steel, or post-consumer high-density polyethylene (HDPE) plastic in its structures. Recycled plastic from a specific source—like recycled milk jugs—is cleaner and safer and carries fewer contaminants than recycled plastics made from electronics. Stainless-steel play sets that have been powder coated to prevent rust are another nontoxic option.

Treated Wood

In addition to its detrimental implications for children when pressure-treated wood is used for play sets and play surfaces, arsenic

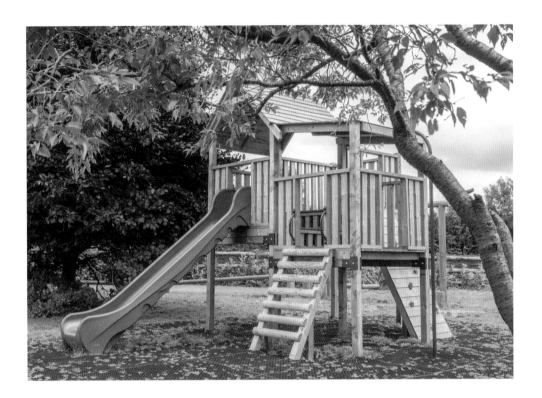

contamination impacts hundreds of millions of people in the world. It is a well-established human carcinogen and has been shown to cause skin, lung, bladder, liver, prostate, and kidney cancers.

Avoid all pressure-treated wood in your yard and home, because even small exposures to arsenic can cause cancer. And CCA-treated wood releases arsenic readily. Pressure-washing a CCA-treated wood deck in your backyard, for example, will release arsenic into the soil and lawn around the deck, creating a carcinogenic hazard that puts your family, pets, and wildlife at risk.

Instead of arsenic-based preservatives, look for nontoxic treatments to protect wood against water and fungal-borne decay. Newly

Nontoxic outdoor toys help children learn through play, setting them up for a lifelong appreciation of the natural world.

developed mineral-based treatments, such as borate, penetrate the outer layers of wood and form a barrier that serves as an effective wood preservative.

If your soil has already been contaminated by arsenic from treated wood runoff, look into soil remediation with mushrooms and mycorrhizae, which can remove and metabolize petroleum products, metals, and agricultural chemicals. Biochar, a highly absorbent natural material that can absorb and sequester toxins from the soil so they can be removed from an area, is another option.

DETOX CLEAN THE YARD AND GARDEN

AFTER YOU REMOVE TOXINS from your yard and garden, it's time to consider the air quality, soil, grass, and play areas.

Air

The air quality of our outdoor spaces needs consideration, as there are so many airborne toxins created by our homes and the homes of others. If you smell smoke from a neighbor's burn pile, you might approach them and make sure they aren't burning wet material, which does not burn well and creates a lot of PAHs. If they're burning garbage, there's a high risk of serious air pollution coming your way. Talk with them about the risks and ask that they take their garbage to the dump instead of burning it. Burning garbage is illegal in many cities and some rural areas, so call for backup if needed.

Although citronella candles and insect-repelling incense are popular for outdoor use, the VOC exposure is risky. Essential oils are a safer insect repellent.

If you smell plastic outdoors, find the source. It could be from the hose, tarps, or toys. Replace these items.

Lawn

Using organic gardening practices will help your lawn stay healthy. Consider letting weeds grow and flower to provide food for bees. You might even consider using your lawn space to grow herbs and a vegetable garden. If you have a lawn where animals play, whether pets or wildlife such as deer, there may be ticks or fleas present. Scatter diatomaceous earth over the lawn every two weeks to kill them through desiccation. The powder will wash into the soil once it rains; if you live in a dry area, you can sprinkle the area with water to help the diatomaceous earth penetrate the soil.

Soil

If chemicals such as pesticides or herbicides have been used in your soil, you can remediate to remove these toxic compounds. Mycoremediation—using mushroom spores that break down chemicals—is one option. Research suggests that mushrooms can convert pesticides and herbicides to more innocuous compounds, remove heavy metals, and break down plastic. Biochar can be used to clean up heavy metals in the soil. Once your soil is cleaned up, add an organic mycorrhizae product to support healthy soil, nourish plants, and produce lush growth.

Concrete

Pressure-wash concrete on your property to remove oil stains, moss, and mold. Spray with Tea Tree Wash. Concrete is porous, and the tea tree essential oil will penetrate deeply for a longer-lasting clean by killing embedded mold and moss.

Wood Decking

If your deck needs to be washed—whether it's stained, treated, or oiled—try this solution: Mix 4 cups warm water, 1 tablespoon Sal Suds, and 1 teaspoon tea tree essential oil. Apply the solution to your deck by dipping a cloth into the bowl of sudsy water and wiping the surfaces. If needed, use a scrub brush, and then rinse with a hose or wipe down with a damp cloth. Pressure washing is not advised for wood decking because it can damage treatments such as paint, stain, and oil, often leading to an expensive repair job. The wood will also rot much faster without paint, stain, or oil. Pressure washers also flush out preservative treatments that may contain chromium, copper, and arsenic and leach them into the soil, where there is risk of human and animal exposures.

Home Entryways

If you are concerned about pests such as ants, ground bees, and mice entering your home, garage, or shed, drip full-strength tea tree or peppermint essential oil along the door thresholds, in the soil under windowsills, and any other entries such as crawl space doors. Avoid painted surfaces as it will cause damage to the paint. Many creatures find the strong smell of essential oils intolerable. Reapply every few weeks if you live in a rainy area and at least once a month if you live in a dry area. You will likely find that there is no need for traps or poisons.

THAT'S IT!

Your outdoor areas are safer and hopefully more enjoyable now that you can relax and use every part of your yard to play, garden, and enjoy the wildlife.

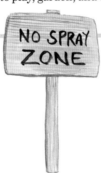

YOUR NONTOXIC LIFESTYLE

YOU NOW HAVE THE INSIGHTS and information you need for staying healthy by avoiding exposures to some of the most common disease-causing toxins in daily life. You also have a trained eye, so you can see toxins and potential sources of illness where others are unaware. Spread the word, educate your friends and family, and stay the course. Enjoy your truly clean home—a transformation you have made through your effort and diligence. I hope that your home detox has enhanced your health, and that you are feeling the benefits of living a nontoxic life. Your passion for healthy living is a beautiful thing for society as a whole; and if kids live in your house, know that you are supporting their health today and into the future, and this means healthier humans for generations to come.

   You are not alone in your new toxin-free lifestyle. When challenges and situations arise, I am here to help you stay on track. Please visit my website **daniellachace.com** for up-to-date resources, to keep in touch, and to further expand wellness in your home.

GLOSSARY

ACETALDEHYDE. A reactive product made from ethanol that is used to help combine chemicals in the production of perfumes, drugs, and dyes.

ACETONE. Also known as propanone. A pungent compound used as a solvent in nail polish remover, lacquer, varnish, waxes, paint remover, polishes, particleboard, and some upholstery fabrics.

ACROLEIN. Also known as propenal. An aldehyde that smells like burned fat, it is used to kill weeds, and it contributes to air pollution.

ACRYLAMIDE. A chemical that can form in some foods during high-temperature cooking, such as frying, roasting, and baking; for example, french fries and potato chips have measurable acrylamide levels. It is also found in cigarette smoke and e-cigarette vapors.

ACRYLIC. A synthetic material (plastic, fabric, fiber, or paint) made from acrylic acid.

AEROSOL. A spray and suspension of fine solid or liquid particles, such as dust, smoke, or mist.

ALDEHYDES. One of a group of highly reactive organic compounds with a strong odor. They are used in many fragranced products. The most well known is formaldehyde.

ALKYLBENZENE SULFONATE. Also known as benzenesulfonic acid. A synthetic compound used as a surfactant in personal care products and in household products including laundry detergent and spray cleaners.

ALKYLPHENOL. One of a family of organic compounds made by the alkylation of phenols and found in many synthetic surfactants, cleaning products, pesticides, and plastics. They are also found in personal care products, especially hair products and lubricants, and are active components of many spermicides.

AMMONIA. A compound of nitrogen and hydrogen. Its gas has a characteristic pungent smell. It is used in many household products, including floor polishing waxes, furniture polish, and cleaning solutions.

ANTIMONY TRIOXIDE. A chemical used in the manufacture of some polyethylene terephthalate (PET) plastic, which is used to make food and beverage containers. It is mainly used as a flame retardant in products such as memory foam.

ASTRINGENT. A chemical that shrinks or constricts body tissues.

BENZENE. A solvent that is among the most utilized chemicals in the United States. It is found in jet fuel, diesel fuel, and gasoline and used in paints, lacquers, varnish removers, industrial solvents, paint thinners, industrial cleaning and degreasing formulations, polystyrene, detergents, drugs, and pesticides.

BENZYL BUTYL PHTHALATE (BBP). A phthalate used as a plasticizer for PVC, vinyl foams, perfumes, hair sprays, adhesives, glues, automotive products, vinyl floor coverings, artificial leather, and children's toys.

BIOCIDE. Any chemical compound or microorganism, whether synthetic or natural, that destroys, deters, renders harmless, or exerts a controlling effect on any other organism. Pesticides, fungicides, and herbicides are all biocides.

BIODEGRADABLE. Capable of being decomposed by water, oxygen, as well as bacteria or other living organisms.

BISPHENOL A (BPA). A chemical used in the production of polycarbonate plastics and epoxy resins. Although restricted due to the health hazards it poses, it is still one of the most common chemicals produced by the plastics industry and used for food and drink packaging, infant bottles, medical devices, and more.

BLEACH. See *sodium hypochlorite*.

BROMINATED. Containing bromine.

BROMINATED FLAME RETARDANTS (BFRs). Man-made chemicals added to products to make them less flammable, used commonly in plastics, textiles, and electronics. BFRs belong to a large group of organic halogen chemical compounds. They are highly persistent and build up in the environment and in our bodies. They cause adverse effects in humans and wildlife. Although some BFRs have been banned or voluntarily withdrawn from usage by manufacturers, existing and new BFR formulas continue to be used.

BROMINE. A chemical element in the halide family that is similar to chlorine. It is commonly used in flame retardants and baked goods and for water sanitation in pools and spas.

BUTOXYETHANOL. Also known as 2-butoxyethanol (2-BE), butyl cellosolve, and ethylene glycol monobutyl ether (EGBE). A butyl ether of ethylene glycol that is a solvent for paints and surface coatings, cleaning products, and many other applications. It is also approved by the FDA to be used in processed food as an antimicrobial, defoamer, stabilizer, and adhesive agent.

CARBON DISULFIDE. A toxic flammable liquid used as a solvent in the making of products including rubber, viscose, rayon, and cellophane.

CARBON MONOXIDE (CO). A highly toxic, odorless, flammable gas. Present in exhaust gases from petrol (gas) engines and furnaces.

CHLORINE. A powerful oxidizer and an active agent in many household bleaches. Since pure chlorine is a toxic corrosive gas, these products usually also contain hypochlorite, which releases chlorine slowly.

COAL TAR. A liquid made by a process of distillation of coal with chemical solvents. Due to its black color, it is used in cosmetics.

DI(2-ETHYLHEXYL) PHTHALATE (DEHP). Also known as bis(2-ethylhexyl) phthalate, diethylhexyl phthalate, and dioctyl phthalate (DOP). A common phthalate used as a plasticizer for PVC, in many household items, and as a fragrance carrier in cosmetics, personal care products, laundry detergents, colognes, scented candles, and air fresheners.

DIBUTYL PHTHALATE (DBP). Also known as di-n-butyl phthalate. An oily liquid phthalate added to some plastics to make them flexible, including some wire and cable insulation, gloves, tubing, garden hoses, and shoes. It is also used in personal care products, perfumes, nail polishes, and rocket fuel.

DIETHANOLAMINE (DEA). This liquid chemical compound is used in industry in metalworking and die-casting and in household and personal care products as an emulsifier to produce foam. It can be found in detergents, shampoo, toothpaste, lotion, and deodorant.

DIETHYLENE GLYCOL (DEG). A compound chemical liquid used as a solvent and as an antifreeze solution. Found in brake fluid, cigarettes, and some dyes.

DIETHYLENE GLYCOL MONOMETHYL ETHER (DEGME). Also known as 2-(2-methoxyethoxy) ethanol and methoxydiglycol. A solvent used for dyes, nitrocellulose, paints, inks, resins, and stains, among other applications.

DIISOCYANATE. A family of reactive compounds used for making resins, plastics, and polyurethane products such as memory foam. Found in products including cushioning for furniture, mattresses, footwear, car interiors, carpet underlay, and packaging.

DIISONONYL PHTHALATE (DINP). A phthalate used as a plasticizer to make plastic consumer products, including some polyvinyl chloride (PVC), vinyl flooring, automobile interiors, wire and cable insulation, gloves, tubing, garden hoses, and shoes.

DIOXANE. Also known as 1,4-dioxane. A solvent used to stabilize chlorinated solvents and in resins, oils, waxes, some dyes, and certain fumigants, deodorants, and preservatives. It is a contaminant in cosmetics, detergents, and shampoos.

DIOXIN. Dioxins are by-products of manufacturing processes including smelting, chlorine bleaching, and the production of herbicides and pesticides.

ENDOCRINE DISRUPTING CHEMICAL (EDC). Manufactured substance that inadvertently interrupts the endocrine system and hormones.

EPIGENETICS. Genetic alterations that involve DNA methylation through exposures to particular triggers, such as hormones, toxins, and nutrients.

ESTERS. Chemical compounds used as solvents for a broad array of plastics, plasticizers, resins, and lacquers.

ESTROGENIC ACTIVITY. Activity that mimics or interrupts natural estrogen activity.

ETHANOL. A simple alcohol and natural by-product of plant fermentation. It is used as a preservative in lotions and hairspray, an antimicrobial in hand sanitizers, and a solvent in paints and varnish, among other applications. Found in a wide range of products including personal care, paints, varnishes, and fuel.

ETHANOLAMINE. Also known as 2-aminoethanol or monoethanolamine (MEA). A compound used in detergents, emulsifiers, polishes, pharmaceuticals, corrosion inhibitors, and cosmetics.

ETHOXYLATE. A synthetic compound used as a wetting and cleaning agent in cosmetics, agriculture, textile, paper, oil, and various other process industries. Used in cleaning products for removing fatty substances from synthetic fibers and hard surfaces.

ETHYL ACETATE. A colorless volatile liquid with a fruity smell, used as a plastics solvent and in flavorings and perfumes. Also used in place of methyl ethyl ketone as the main solvent in acetone-free nail polish remover products.

ETHYLENE GLYCOL. Similar in structure and use to diethylene glycol, these chemical compounds are used to make antifreeze, polyester fibers, car wash fluids, deicing products, vehicle brake fluids, industrial solvents, paints, and cosmetics.

ETHYLENE GLYCOL MONOMETHYL ETHER (EGME). Also known as 2-methoxyethanol or methyl cellosolve. A solvent used for many different purposes, such as varnishes, dyes, and resins, and as an additive in airplane deicing solutions and leather dyes and as a sealing agent.

FLAME RETARDANT. A material that prevents the start of or slows the growth of a fire.

FLUORIDE. A halide element made from the reduction of the element fluorine. Used in fluoridation of drinking water and in the manufacture of dental preparations such as toothpaste, mouthwashes, and teeth whitening solutions. It is also used in the production of steel, aluminum, glass and enamel, and insecticides and as a preservative for glues and wood.

FLUOROPOLYMER. A class of fluorocarbon-based polymers, meaning they have many carbon-fluorine bonds, within the group of per- and polyfluoroalkyl substances.

FORMALDEHYDE. A chemical used as an industrial disinfectant and as a preservative. It is commonly used in pressed-wood products, such as particleboard, plywood, and fiberboard; glues and adhesives; permanent-press fabrics; paper product coatings; in medicines and cosmetics; and in certain insulation materials.

GLYCOL. Any of a class of organic compounds belonging to the alcohol family.

GLYCOL ETHER. One of a group of solvents based on alkyl ethers of either ethylene glycol or propylene glycol. They are used in glass, carpet, flooring, paints, pharmaceuticals, sunscreens, cosmetics, inks, dyes, degreasers, aerosol paints, and adhesives. They are absorbed as volatile fumes from the air by the skin as well as through inhalation.

HALOACETIC ACIDS (HAAs). Chemical compounds that contain chlorine and bromine. They are formed by the reaction of disinfectants (chlorine, chloramine, chlorine dioxide, and ozone) with natural organic matter and bromide.

HAZARDOUS AIR POLLUTANTS (HAPs). Air pollutants known to have serious health impacts.

HAZARDOUS WASTE. Any waste that carries substantial or potential threat to public health or the environment.

HEAVY METALS. Natural metallic elements with a high density that are used in manufactured products and are toxic even in low concentrations. They include aluminum, antimony, arsenic, barium, bismuth, boron, cadmium, molybdenum, nickel, and tin.

HEPA FILTER. High-efficiency particulate air filter. This is a type of pleated mechanical air filter that captures a high percentage of dust, pollen, mold, bacteria, and airborne particles.

HEXANE. A solvent used in gasoline; in glues for shoes, leather products, and roofing; for degreasing; and in textile manufacturing. It is also used in food-based canola oil, soybean oil, and soy food products.

HYDANTOIN. An antimicrobial formaldehyde preservative with the trade name Glydant that is found in products like shampoos, hair conditioners, hair gels, and skin care products.

HYDROCARBON. A class of chemical compounds composed only of the elements carbon and hydrogen. Hydrocarbons are the principal constituents of petroleum and natural gas. They serve as fuels and lubricants as well as raw materials to produce plastics, fibers, rubbers, solvents, explosives, and industrial chemicals.

HYDROFLUORIC ACID. Also known as hydrogen fluoride. A gas used in pharmaceutical antidepressant medications such as fluoxetine (Prozac) and in polytetrafluoroethylene (Teflon). It is also used in the production of refrigerants, herbicides, pharmaceuticals, high-octane gasoline, plastics, electrical components, and fluorescent lightbulbs.

ISOCYANATE. One of a family of chemicals used in the production of many polyurethane products. They are increasingly used in the automobile industry for auto body repair and building insulation materials.

ISOPROPYL ALCOHOL. Also known as propan-2-ol, isopropanol, and 2-propanol. A synthetic alcohol used in personal care products, including aftershave lotions, hand lotions, and cosmetics.

LIQUID CARBON DIOXIDE. The liquid form of a significant greenhouse gas linked to global warming. Liquid carbon dioxide is used as a refrigerant, in fire extinguishers, for inflating life rafts and life jackets, in blasting coal, in foaming rubber and plastics, for immobilizing animals before slaughter, and in carbonated beverages.

MAMMARY TOXICANT. Any substance that is toxic to breast cells, such as aluminum and plastics, and especially those that are breast cell carcinogens.

MELAMINE. Also known as cyanuramide and triaminotriazine. A synthetic resin made from dicyandiamide, hydrogen cyanide, or urea that is molded into dishes, containers, utensils, and handles and used as a laminating agent and coating material for wood, paper, and textiles.

METHYLENE CHLORIDE. Also known as dichloromethane. A halogen compound used as a solvent in paint-stripping formulations, as a degreaser in automotive products, and in metal airplane and railroad components. It is also used for extraction in food and beverage products; for example, it is used to remove caffeine from unroasted coffee beans and tea leaves to make decaffeinated coffee and tea.

METHYL ETHYL KETONE (MEK). Also known as 2-butanone. A solvent used in nail polish remover.

MICROPLASTICS. Small plastic pieces that are less than 5 millimeters.

NANOPARTICLES. Very small particles ranging between 1 and 100 nanometers. To compare, a human hair is approximately 80,000 to 100,000 nanometers wide. Undetectable by the human eye, nanoparticles from household products or cosmetics, for example, can cross the blood-brain barrier and be easily absorbed through the skin and the lungs.

NANOPLASTICS. Small plastic particles that are less than 100 nanometers.

NAPTHAS. Petroleum products. Chemicals used as solvents and dilutants used as a paint thinner and cleaning agent and in the manufacture of plastic.

NAPHTHALENE. A compound made from coal tar that is used in mothballs, moth flakes, white tar, and tar camphor. When mixed with air, naphthalene vapors easily burn, as when tobacco or wood is burned.

NEUROTOXIN. A substance that alters the structure or function of the nervous system. Neurotoxins in our everyday household products include aluminum, arsenic, benzene, ethanol, lead, and toluene.

OBESOGEN. Something that promotes obesity in individuals or populations. Endocrine-disrupting chemicals (EDCs) are major potential obesogens.

OFF-GAS. To give off or release a gas, especially one emitted as the by-product of a chemical process.

ORGANOPHOSPHATE FLAME RETARDANTS (OPFRs). Additives in plasticizers, foams, hydraulic fluids, antifoam agents, and coatings for electronic components to inhibit flames. OPFRs were developed as an alternative to brominated and chlorinated flame retardants, which have high environmental and health concerns. They are widely used in textiles, furniture, and electronics as plasticizers.

PARABENS. Parahydroxy-benzoates or esters of parahydroxybenzoic acid. Parabens are a group of chemicals widely used as artificial preservatives in cosmetic, body care, and pharmaceutical products since the 1920s. Today they are found in shampoos, conditioners, moisturizers, skin cleansers, sunscreens, deodorants, shaving gels, toothpaste, makeup, and more.

PARADICHLOROBENZENE (PDCB). A chlorinated aromatic hydrocarbon used as a fumigant in insecticides, bug repellents, and mildew treatment.

PERCHLOROETHYLENE. Also known as perc or tetrachloroethylene. A colorless toxic liquid used as a solvent in dry cleaning, to remove grease from metals, and in consumer products including paint strippers, spot removers, and aerosol preparations. It has also been detected in drinking water supplies from contaminated groundwater sources.

PERFLUOROOCTANOIC ACID (PFOA). A type of per- and polyfluoroalkyl substance used to manufacture certain polymers, such as nonstick coatings on cooking pans.

PERSISTENT ENVIRONMENTAL POLLUTANTS (POPs). Chemicals and synthetic compounds that do not biodegrade and stay in the environment for periods up to hundreds of years.

PHOSPHATE. A chemical compound that contains the mineral phosphorus. Phosphates are often used in fertilizers, flame retardants, and detergents.

PHTHALATES. A family of chemical compounds primarily used to make polyvinyl chloride (PVC) because they make vinyl flexible and pliant. They are used in many products, including flooring, adhesives, personal care products, clothing, and food packaging. Large amounts of phthalate particulates are found in household dust and even in rain. Phthalates are the single most common man-made product in the world.

PLASTICIZER. A substance that is added to a material to make it softer and more flexible, to decrease its viscosity, or to decrease friction during its handling in manufacture.

POLYAMIDE. A plastic polymer, also known as nylon, that is used in synthetic fibers, car interiors, carpets, kitchen utensils, and sportswear.

POLYBROMINATED DIPHENYL ETHER (PBDE). A class of brominated compounds used as flame retardants in many products, including TVs, toasters, mattresses, and drapes. In recent years, PBDEs have generated international concern over their widespread distribution in the environment, their potential to bioaccumulate in humans, and their adverse health effects.

POLYCYCLIC AROMATIC HYDROCARBON (PAH). One of a group of hydrocarbons that are persistent and bioaccumulate. Exposure usually occurs by breathing smoke or by eating grilled foods. Some PAHs have been identified as carcinogenic, mutagenic, and teratogenic.

POLYESTER. A synthetic resin used to make textiles. Polyester fabrics are used extensively in apparel and home furnishings, from shirts and pants to bedding and upholstered furniture.

POLYETHYLENE. A synthetic resin made from ethylene gas that is used to produce plastic bags, food containers, and other packaging.

POLYETHYLENE GLYCOL. A synthetic resin made from ethylene glycol that is used mainly as a solvent or wax.

POLYFLUOROALKYL SUBSTANCES (PFAS). Also known as perfluorinated chemicals, these are used to make products resistant to stains, grease, and water and to reduce friction. They are perhaps best known for their use in making nonstick coatings for pans, but they are also used in fabrics, carpets, fast-food packaging, floor polishes, denture cleaners, and shampoos, among other things.

POLYPROPYLENE. A synthetic resin made from propylene, used for ropes, fabrics, and molded objects.

POLYTETRAFLUORO-ETHYLENE (PTFE). A synthetic fluoropolymer used as a resin to coat cookware, gaskets, seals, and hoses. The most common example is Teflon.

POLYURETHANE. A synthetic resin used for, among other things, padding and insulation in furniture, clothing, and packaging and in the manufacture of adhesives, elastomers (elastic polymers), and fillers.

POLYVINYL CHLORIDE (PVC). The common synthetic plastic polymer used to make pipes, doors, windows, bottles, packaging, food-covering sheets, leather, flooring, inflatable products, personal care tools, and more.

PROPYLENE GLYCOL. A liquid alcohol that is used as a solvent in antifreeze, plastics, and perfume. Commonly used as a food additive to preserve moisture as well as dissolve colors and flavors. It is also used in many personal care products, medications, and cosmetics.

QUATERNARY AMMONIUM COMPOUNDS. Also known as quats, these are a group of chemical salts used for a variety of purposes including as preservatives, surfactants, and antistatic agents and as disinfectants and sanitizers.

SODIUM BORATE. Also known as borax, this is a compound made from the mineral boron and a salt of boric acid. Powdered borax is white, consisting of soft colorless crystals that dissolve in water. It is used in many detergents, cosmetics, and enamel glazes.

SODIUM HYDROXIDE. A highly caustic alkali that decomposes proteins and may cause severe chemical burns. It is used in the manufacture of paper, textiles, soaps, detergents, and drain cleaners. It is also used in the treatment of drinking water to raise the pH of the water to a level that minimizes the corrosion of lead pipes.

SODIUM HYPOCHLORITE. Also known as liquid bleach (when in solution). The household chemical widely used as a disinfectant and whitening agent.

SODIUM LAURETH SULFATE (SLES). Also known as lauryl ether sulfate. A compound added to personal care and cleaning products and herbicides as a surfactant. It is made from either petroleum or plant oils such as coconut or palm kernel.

SODIUM LAURYL SULFATE (SLS). Also known as sodium laurilsulfate or sodium dodecyl sulfate. A compound used as a surfactant in many cleaning and hygiene products. It can be made from petroleum or from plant oils such as coconut or palm kernel.

SOLVENT. A substance that dissolves another substance, such as paint thinner.

TALC. Also known as talcum powder. Magnesium silicate powder, which has been used as a cosmetic due to its ability to wick moisture.

TERPENE. One of a group of aromatic compounds that create the characteristic scent of many plants, such as cannabis, pine, and lavender.

THYMOL. An antimicrobial compound present in the essential oil of thyme and used as a flavoring and preservative.

TOLUENE. Also known as methylbenzene. A volatile organic compound used in paint thinners, paints, nail polish, lacquers, adhesives, and rubber, among other applications.

TRICHLOROETHYLENE (TCE). A chemical solvent used to remove grease from metal parts. It is also an ingredient in adhesives, paint removers, and stain removers.

TRICLOCARBAN (TCC). An antibacterial and antifungal that is similar to triclosan in structure and use.

TRICLOSAN (TCS). Also known as 2,4,4-trichloro-2-hydroxydiphenyl ether, trichloro-2-hydroxydiphenyl ether, and 5-chloro-(2,4-dichlorophenoxy) phenol. An antibacterial and antifungal agent present in many consumer products, including toothpaste, soaps, deodorant, detergents, and toys.

TRIETHANOLAMINE (TEA). An amine that is derived from the petroleum industry and made with ammonia. It is used in the making of surfactants for cosmetics and medications.

VINYL. A type of plastic made from synthetic resin and polyvinyl chloride.

VOLATILE ORGANIC COMPOUNDS (VOCs). Gases emitted into the air from certain solids, liquids, or processes.

XYLENE. A petrochemical used as a solvent in the manufacturing of chemicals, agricultural sprays, adhesives, and coatings. It is an ingredient in aviation fuel, gasoline, paint thinners, and more.

FURTHER READING

Clean Green: Tips and Recipes for a Naturally Clean, More Sustainable Home by Jen Chillingsworth (Hardie Grant Quadrille, 2020).

Detox Your Home: A Guide to Removing Toxins from Your Life and Bringing Health into Your Home by Christine Dimmick (Rowman & Littlefield, 2018).

Entangled Life: How Fungi Make Our Worlds, Change Our Minds & Shape Our Futures by Merlin Sheldrake (Random House, 2021).

Mycelium Running: How Mushrooms Can Help Save the World by Paul Stamets (Ten Speed Press, 2005).

Never Home Alone: From Microbes to Millipedes, Camel Crickets, and Honeybees, the Natural History of Where We Live by Rob Dunn (Basic Books, 2018).

New Minimalism: Decluttering and Design for Sustainable, Intentional Living by Cary Telander Fortin and Kyle Louise Quilici (Sasquatch Books, 2018).

Plastic-Free: How I Kicked the Plastic Habit and How You Can Too by Beth Terry (Skyhorse, 2012).

Plastic Purge: How to Use Less Plastic, Eat Better, Keep Toxins Out of Your Body and Help Save the Sea Turtles by Micheal SanClements (St. Martin's Griffin, 2014).

Pure Skin Care: Nourishing Recipes for Vibrant Skin & Natural Beauty by Stephanie L. Tourles (Storey, 2018).

Silent Spring by Rachel Carson (Houghton Mifflin, 40th anniversary edition, 2002).

Simply Living Well: A Guide to Creating a Natural, Low-Waste Home by Julia Watkins (Houghton Mifflin Harcourt, 2020).

The Toxin Solution: How Hidden Poisons in the Air, Water, Food, and Products We Use Are Destroying Our Health—and What We Can Do to Fix It by Joseph Pizzorno (HarperOne, 2017).

Toxin Toxout: Getting Harmful Chemicals Out of Our Bodies and Our World by Bruce Lourie and Rick Smith (St. Martin's Griffin, 2014).

Zero Waste Home: The Ultimate Guide to Simplifying Your Life by Reducing Your Waste by Bea Johnson (Scribner, 2013).

RESOURCES

HOME TOXIN TESTING SOURCES AND LABS

EMF Reader
www.radmeters.com
Pocket-sized EMF reader lights up where there are hot spots of electromagnetic energy.

Green Building Supply
www.greenbuildingsupply.com
A trusted source for nontoxic and eco-friendly building materials and lab test kits, including tests for mold, asbestos, water quality, microwave oven leakage, radon, pesticides, lead, and carbon monoxide.

Home Air Check
www.homeaircheck.com
Home air tests for VOCs, mold, formaldehyde, tobacco smoke, and over 500 other compounds and chemicals.

SLGI
www.slabinc.com
Offers air, water, and solid material tests for lead, mercury, hexavalent chromium, asbestos, mold, bacteria, PCBs, and many more toxic compounds.

ONLINE TOXICOLOGY RESOURCES

Agency for Toxic Substances and Disease Registry
www.atsdr.cdc.gov
The US Agency for Toxic Substances and Disease Registry (ATSDR) works to minimize human health risks associated with exposure to hazardous substances.

Beyond Pesticides
www.beyondpesticides.org
This nonprofit network is working to set national pesticide policy by putting pressure on the chemical industry. Their website is a resource for finding natural pest management, bee protection initiatives, tools for communicating with schools, and organic landscape management, among many other wonderful strategies for reducing pesticide use.

Campaign for Safe Cosmetics

www.safecosmetics.org

The Campaign for Safe Cosmetics coalition works to protect the health of consumers, workers, and the environment through public education and engagement, corporate accountability and sustainability campaigns, and legislative advocacy designed to eliminate dangerous chemicals linked to adverse health impacts from cosmetics and personal care products.

Center for Biological Diversity

www.biologicaldiversity.org

This group takes direct action to protect humans and other animals from toxins, save endangered species, and improve environmental health through work in science, law, and media.

Ecology Center

www.ecocenter.org

The Ecology Center is dedicated to testing everyday products for toxicity and publishing safe buying guides to help consumers avoid toxic household materials.

Environmental Health News

www.ehn.org

The EHN is a nonprofit publication on environmental health sciences, covering environmental toxins, health issues, and climate change.

Environmental Working Group

www.ewg.org

The EWG provides detailed research, consumer guides, and product ratings, as well as nontoxic recommendations for products. If you question whether an ingredient in a product is toxic, this is one of the most comprehensive sites for getting answers.

National Library of Medicine

www.nlm.nih.gov

The National Library of Medicine is part of the US National Institutes of Health and offers a search engine for medical, environmental medicine, toxicology, and health journals around the world.

PLOS ONE

https://journals.plos.org/plosone

This inclusive journal community publishes multidisciplinary and interdisciplinary research covering over 200 subject areas across science, engineering, medicine, and the related social sciences and humanities.

PubChem

https://pubchem.ncbi.nlm.nih.gov

The National Library of Medicine provides PubChem, which includes ToxNet, a database of studies on toxins.

PubMed

www.pubmed.gov

PubMed is a portal to the National Institutes of Health and its free biomedical literature search engine that provides access to more than 27 million articles. This is an easy system to use to search specific health conditions and toxins.

Silent Spring Institute

https://silentspring.org

This group works to uncover the environmental causes of breast cancer. Their website provides good information about carcinogens, and they work toward large policy changes to protect human health.

Toxic-Free Future

https://toxicfreefuture.org

This group conducts research and advocacy to win strong health protections for people and the environment.

BIBLIOGRAPHY

CHAPTER ONE: THE HOME DETOX METHOD

Ammonia
Dasarathy S, et al. 2017. Ammonia toxicity: from head to toe?. *Metabolic Brain Disease*.

Bleach
Casas L, et al. 2015. Domestic use of bleach and infections in children: a multicentre cross-sectional study. *Occupational and Environmental Medicine*.

Kawalilak LT, Fransson BA, Alessio TL. 2017. Management of a facial partial thickness chemical burn in a dog caused by bleach. *Journal of Veterinary Emergency and Critical Care*.

Matulonga B, et al. 2016. Women using bleach for home cleaning are at increased risk of non-allergic asthma. *Respiratory Medicine*.

Morim A, Guldner GT. 2019. Chlorine gas toxicity. StatPearls.

Peck B, et al. 2011. Spectrum of sodium hypochlorite toxicity in man—also a concern for nephrologists. *NDT Plus*.

Carpet Cleaners
Berg NW, et al. 2018. Safety assessment of the use of *Bacillus*-based cleaning products. *Food and Chemical Toxicology*.

Sanz-Gallen P, et al. 2019. Perchloroethylene: acute occupational poisoning and a proposal for its replacement with other less toxic substances. *Medycyna Pracy*.

Volney G, et al. 2018. Naphthalene toxicity: methemoglobinemia and acute intravascular hemolysis. *Cureus*.

Cleaners
Bondi CA, et al. 2015. Human and environmental toxicity of sodium lauryl sulfate (SLS): evidence for safe use in household cleaning products. *Environmental Health Insights*.

Paciência I, et al. 2019. Exposure to indoor endocrine-disrupting chemicals and childhood asthma and obesity. *Allergy*.

Slaughter RJ, et al. 2019. The clinical toxicology of sodium hypochlorite. *Clinical Toxicology*.

Degreaser
Bagchi G, Waxman DJ. 2008. Toxicity of ethylene glycol monomethyl ether: impact on testicular gene expression. *International Journal of Andrology*.

Gerster FM, et al. 2014. Hazardous substances in frequently used professional cleaning products. *International Journal of Occupational and Environmental Health*.

Dishwasher Detergent
O'Donnell KA. 2017. Pediatric toxicology: household product ingestions. *Pediatric Annals*.

Quail MT. 2018. Preventing laundry detergent pod toxicity. *Nursing*.

Sjogren PP, Skarda DE, Park AH. 2017. Upper aerodigestive injuries from detergent ingestion in children. *The Laryngoscope*.

Drain Cleaner
Al-Busaidi AS, et al. 2019. Cutaneous drain opener burns: report from a tertiary care burns unit. *Burns Open*.

Boonekamp C, Voruz F, Fehlmann C. 2018. Accidental aspiration of a solid tablet of sodium hydroxide. *BMJ Case Reports*.

Dry Cleaners
Lash LH. 2019. Environmental and genetic factors influencing kidney toxicity. *Seminars in Nephrology*.

Essential Oils
Gemeda N, et al. 2018. Development, characterization, and evaluation of novel broad-spectrum antimicrobial topical formulations from *Cymbopogon martini* (Roxb.) W. Watson essential oil. *Evidence-Based Complementary and Alternative Medicine*.

Nazzaro F, et al. 2017. Essential oils and antifungal activity. *Pharmaceuticals*.

Stringaro A, Colone M, Angiolella L. 2018. Antioxidant, antifungal, antibiofilm, and cytotoxic activities of *Mentha* spp. essential oils. *Medicines*.

Ethylene Glycol
Amoroso L, et al. 2017. Ethylene glycol toxicity: a retrospective pathological study in cats. *Veterinaria Italiana*.

Flame Retardants
Gibson EA, et al. 2018. Flame retardant exposure assessment: findings from a behavioral intervention study. *Journal of Exposure Science & Environmental Epidemiology*.

Jones M, et al. 2018. Thermal degradation and fire properties of fungal mycelium and mycelium-biomass composite materials. *Scientific Reports*.

Lash LH. 2019. Environmental and genetic factors influencing kidney toxicity. *Seminars in Nephrology*.

Flea Treatments
Boffetta P, Desai V. 2018. Exposure to permethrin and cancer risk: a systematic review. *Critical Reviews in Toxicology*.

Rust MK. 2017. The biology and ecology of cat fleas and advancements in their pest management: a review. *Insects*.

Skolarczyk J, Pekar J, Nieradko-Iwanicka B. 2017. Immune disorders induced by exposure to pyrethroid insecticides. *Postępy Higieny i Medycyny Doświadczalnej*.

Furniture Polish
Tormoehlen LM, Tekulve KJ, Naagas KA. 2014. Hydrocarbon toxicity: a review. *Clinical Toxicology*.

Glass Cleaner
Almulhim KN. 2017. Fatal butane toxicity and delayed onset of refractory ventricular fibrillation. *Saudi Medical Journal*.

Paciência I, et al. 2019. Exposure to indoor endocrine-disrupting chemicals and childhood asthma and obesity. *Allergy*.

Hair Salons
Gera R, et al. 2018. Does the use of hair dyes increase the risk of developing breast cancer? A meta-analysis and review of the literature. *Anticancer Research*.

Vitale CM, Gutovitz S. 2019. Aromatic (benzene, toluene) toxicity. StatPearls.

Mold
Becher R, et al. 2017. Dampness and moisture problems in Norwegian homes. *International Journal of Environmental Research and Public Health*.

Nazzaro F, et al. 2017. Essential oils and antifungal activity. *Pharmaceuticals*.

Multipurpose Cleaners
Casas L, et al. 2013. Use of household cleaning products, exhaled nitric oxide and lung function in children. *The European Respiratory Journal*.

Peshin SS, Gupta YK. 2018. Poisoning due to household products: a ten years retrospective analysis of telephone calls to the National Poisons Information Centre, All India Institute of Medical Sciences, New Delhi, India. *Journal of Forensic and Legal Medicine*.

Slaughter RJ, et al. 2019. The clinical toxicology of sodium hypochlorite. *Clinical Toxicology*.

Nail Salons
Felzenszwalb I, et al. 2019. Toxicological evaluation of nail polish waste discarded in the environment. *Environmental Science and Pollution Research*.

Young AS, et al. 2018. Phthalate and organophosphate plasticizers in nail polish: evaluation of labels and ingredients. *Environmental Science & Technology*.

Oven Cleaners
Day RC, et al. 2017. Toxicity resulting from exposure to oven cleaners as reported to the UK National Poisons Information Service (NPIS) from 2009 to 2015. *Clinical Toxicology*.

Hashmi MU, et al. 2018. Clinico-epidemiological characteristics of corrosive ingestion: a cross-sectional study at a tertiary care hospital of Multan, South-Punjab Pakistan. *Cureus*.

Pet Bedding
Benzoni T, Hatcher JD. 2018. Bleach toxicity. *Journal of the American Association of Laboratory Animal Sciences*.

Yang H, et al. 2018. A common antimicrobial additive increases colonic inflammation and colitis-associated colon tumorigenesis in mice. *Science Translational Medicine*.

Plastic Food Containers
Dhillon GS, et al. 2015. Triclosan: current status, occurrence, environmental risks and bioaccumulation potential. *International Journal of Environmental Research and Public Health*.

Galloway TS, et al. 2018. An engaged research study to assess the effect of a "real-world" dietary intervention on urinary bisphenol A (BPA) levels in teenagers. *BMJ Open*.

Rastkari N, et al. 2018. Effect of sunlight exposure on phthalates migration from plastic containers to packaged juices. *Journal of Environmental Health Science & Engineering*.

Sponges
Bondi CA, et al. 2015. Human and environmental toxicity of sodium lauryl sulfate (SLS): evidence for safe use in household cleaning products. *Environmental Health Insights*.

Styrofoam Food Containers
Guyton KZ, et al. 2018. Carcinogenicity of styrene. *Environmental Health Perspectives*.

Schaider LA, et al. 2017. Fluorinated compounds in U.S. fast food packaging. *Environmental Science & Technology Letters*.

Tile Cleaners
Heard K. 2017. Hydrofluoric acid. *Critical Care Toxicology*.

Toilet Bowl Cleaners
Bajraktarova-Valjakova E, et al. 2018. Hydrofluoric acid: burns and systemic toxicity, protective measures, immediate and hospital medical treatment. *Open Access Macedonian Journal Medical Science*.

Heard K. 2017. Hydrofluoric acid. *Critical Care Toxicology*.

Mughal BB, Fini J-B, Demeneix, BA. 2018. Thyroid-disrupting chemicals and brain development: an update. *Endocrine Connections.*

Schwerin DL, Hatcher JD. 2019. Hydrofluoric acid burns. StatPearls.

Vally H, Misso N. 2012. Adverse reactions to the sulphite additives. *Gastroenterology and Hepatology from Bed to Bench.*

Water
Honeycutt JA, et al. 2017. Effects of water bottle materials and filtration on bisphenol A content in laboratory animal drinking water. *Journal of the American Association for Laboratory Animal Science.*

Mason SA, Welch V, Neratko J. 2018. Synthetic polymer contamination in bottled water. *Frontiers in Chemistry.*

Sanz-Gallen P, et al. 2019. Perchloroethylene: acute occupational poisoning and a proposal for its replacement with other less toxic substances. *Medycyna Pracy.*

Wood Floor Cleaners
Deshayes S, et al. 2017. Alkylphenol and phthalate contamination of all sources of greywater from French households. *Science of the Total Environment.*

Kawakami T, et al. 2017. Analysis of glycols, glycol ethers, and other volatile organic compounds present in household water-based hand pump sprays. *Journal of Environmental Science and Health.*

Yoga Mats
Jo S-H, et al. 2018. Characterization and flux assessment of airborne phthalates released from polyvinyl chloride consumer goods. *Environmental Research.*

CHAPTER TWO: KITCHEN
Aluminum
Colomina MT, Peris-Sampedro F. 2017. Aluminum and Alzheimer's disease. *Advanced Neurobiology.*

Deshwal GK, Panjagari NR, Alam T. 2019. An overview of paper and paper-based food packaging materials: health safety and environmental concerns. *Journal of Food Science and Technology.*

Inan-Eroglu E, Ayaz A. 2018. Is aluminum exposure a risk factor for neurological disorders? *Journal of Research and Medical Science.*

Weidenhamer JD, et al. 2017. Metal exposures from aluminum cookware: an unrecognized public health risk in developing countries. *Science of the Total Environment.*

Cabinets
Herkert NJ, Jahnke JC, Hornbuckle KC. 2018. Emissions of tetrachlorobiphenyls (PCBs 47, 51, and 68) from polymer resin on kitchen cabinets as a non-aroclor source to residential air. *Environmental Science & Technology.*

Ceramics
Fralick M, Thompson A, Mourad O. 2016. Lead toxicity from glazed ceramic cookware. *Canadian Medical Association Journal.*

Mania M, et al. 2018. Exposure assessment to lead, cadmium, zinc and copper released from ceramic and glass wares intended to come into contact with food. *Annals of the National Institute of Hygiene.*

Coffee Pods
Abe Y, et al. 2021. Determination of formaldehyde and acetaldehyde levels in poly(ethylene terephthalate) (PET) bottled mineral water using a simple and rapid analytical method. *Food Chemistry.*

De Toni L, et al. 2017. Phthalates and heavy metals as endocrine disruptors in food: a study on pre-packed coffee products. *Toxicology Reports.*

Cutting Boards
Wu Y, et al. 2017. Adsorption of phthalates on impervious indoor surfaces. *Environmental Science and Technology.*

Dish Soaps
Ley C, et al. 2018. Triclosan and triclocarban exposure, infectious disease symptoms and antibiotic prescription in infants: a community-based randomized intervention. *PLOS ONE.*

Steinemann AC. 2018. Fragranced consumer products: effects on asthmatics. *Air Quality, Atmosphere & Health.*

Yost LJ, et al. 2016. Human health risk assessment of chloroxylenol in liquid hand soap and dishwashing soap used by consumers and health-care professionals. *Regulatory Toxicology and Pharmacology.*

Dishwasher Soaps
McKenzie LB, et al. 2010. Household cleaning product–related injuries treated in US emergency departments in 1990–2006. *Pediatrics.*

Pierce BL, et al. 2019. A missense variant in FTCD affects arsenic metabolism and toxicity phenotypes in Bangladesh. *PLOS Genetics.*

Nonstick Pans
Bevin BE, et al. 2018. Associations between longitudinal serum perfluoroalkyl substance (PFAS) levels and measures of thyroid hormone, kidney function, and body mass index in the Fernald Community Cohort. *Environmental Pollution.*

Choi H, et al. 2018. Perfluorinated compounds in food stimulants after migration from fluorocarbon resin–coated frying pans, baking utensils, and non-stick baking papers on the Korean market. *Food Additives & Contaminants: Part B.*

Hurley S, et al. 2018. Breast cancer risk and serum levels of per- and poly-fluoroalkyl substances: a case-control study nested in the California Teachers Study. *Environmental Health.*

Sajid M, Ilyas M. 2017. PTFE-coated non-stick cookware and toxicity concerns: a perspective. *Environmental Science and Pollution Research International.*

Shimizu T, et al. 2012. Rare disease polymer fume fever. *BMJ Case Reports.*

Plastic Food Packaging

Bakircioglu D, Kurtulus YB, Ucar G. 2011. Determination of some traces metal levels in cheese samples packaged in plastic and tin containers by ICP-OES after dry, wet and microwave digestion. *Food and Chemical Toxicology.*

Li D, Suh S. 2019. Health risks of chemicals in consumer products: a review. *Environment International.*

Liu M, et al. 2019. The occurrence of bisphenol plasticizers in paired dust and urine samples and its association with oxidative stress. *Chemosphere.*

Yang J, et al. 2019. Migration of phthalates from plastic packages to convenience foods and its cumulative health risk assessments. *Food Additives & Contaminants: Part B.*

Plastic Food Storage Bags

Konieczna A, Rutkowska A, Rachoń D. 2015. Health risk of exposure to bisphenol A (BPA). *Annals of National Institute of Hygiene.*

Plastic Food Storage Containers

Dobrzyńska MM. 2016. Phthalates: widespread occurrence and the effect on male gametes. Part 1. General characteristics, sources and human exposure. *Roczniki Państwowego Zakładu Higieny.*

Groh KJ, et al. 2019. Overview of known plastic packaging–associated chemicals and their hazards. *Science of the Total Environment.*

Yang CZ, et al. 2011. Most plastic products release estrogenic chemicals: a potential health problem that can be solved. *Environmental Health Perspectives.*

Plastic Tableware

Lu Y, et al. 2017. A review of methods for detecting melamine in food samples. *Critical Reviews in Analytical Chemistry.*

Lund KH, Petersen JH. 2006. Migration of formaldehyde and melamine monomers from kitchen- and tableware made of melamine plastic. *Food Additives and Contamination.*

Plastic/Nylon Utensils

Kuang J, Abdallah MA, Harrad S. 2018. Brominated flame retardants in black plastic kitchen utensils: concentrations and human exposure implications. *Science of the Total Environment.*

Olchowik-Grabarek E, et al. 2018. Comparative analysis of BPA and HQ toxic impacts on human erythrocytes, protective effect mechanism of tannins (*Rhus typhina*). *Environmental Science and Pollution Research International.*

Zhan F, et al. 2019. Release and transformation of BTBPE during the thermal treatment of flame retardant ABS plastics. *Environmental Science & Technology.*

Sponges

Cardinale M, et al. 2017. Microbiome analysis and confocal microscopy of used kitchen sponges reveal massive colonization by *Acinetobacter, Moraxella* and *Chryseobacterium* species. *Scientific Reports.*

Weatherly LM, Gosse JA. 2017. Triclosan exposure, transformation, and human health effects. *Journal of Toxicology and Environmental Health, Part B, Critical Reviews.*

Water

Bexfield LM, et al. 2019. Hormones and pharmaceuticals in groundwater used as a source of drinking water across the United States. *Environmental Science & Technology.*

Chen AYY, Olsen T. 2016. Chromated copper arsenate– treated wood: a potential source of arsenic exposure and toxicity in dermatology. *International Journal of Women's Dermatology.*

Jarvis P, et al. 2018. Intake of lead (Pb) from tap water of homes with leaded and low lead plumbing systems. *Science of the Total Environment.*

Kaali S, et al. 2018. Prenatal household air pollution alters cord blood mononuclear cell mitochondrial DNA copy number: sex-specific associations. *International Journal of Environmental Research and Public Health.*

Pierce BL, et al. 2019. A missense variant in *FTCD* is associated with arsenic metabolism and toxicity phenotypes in Bangladesh. *PLOS Genetics.*

Soza-Ried C, et al. 2019. Oncogenic role of arsenic exposure in lung cancer: a forgotten risk factor. *Critical Review Oncology/Hematology.*

Yuan T, et al. 2018. Association between lung cancer risk and inorganic arsenic concentration in drinking water: a dose–response meta-analysis. *Toxicology Research.*

CHAPTER THREE: BATHROOM

Aftershave

Meeker JD, Ferguson K. 2014. Urinary phthalate metabolites are associated with decreased serum testosterone in men, women, and children from NHANES 2011–2012. *Journal of Clinical Endocrinology & Metabolism.*

Nassan FL, et al. 2017. Personal care product use in men and urinary concentrations of select phthalate metabolites and parabens: results from the Environment and Reproductive Health (EARTH) Study. *Environmental Health Perspectives.*

Air Fresheners

ALshaer FI, et al. 2019. Qualitative analysis of air freshener spray. *Journal of Environmental and Public Health.*

Caress SM, Steinemann A. 2009. Prevalence of fragrance sensitivity in the American population. *Journal of Environmental Health.*

Kawakami T, et al. 2017. Analysis of glycols, glycol ethers, and other volatile organic compounds present in household water-based hand pump sprays. *Journal of Environmental Science and Health, Part A, Toxic/Hazardous Substances & Environmental Engineering.*

Kim S, et al. 2015. Characterization of air freshener emission: the potential health effects. *The Journal of Toxicological Sciences.*

Kopelovich L, et al. 2015. Screening-level human health risk assessment of toluene and dibutyl phthalate in nail lacquers. *Food and Chemical Toxicology.*

Silva-Néto RP, Peres MFP, Valença MM. 2014. Odorant substances that trigger headaches in migraine patients. *Cephalalgia.*

Snyder R. 2012. Leukemia and benzene. *International Journal of Environmental Research and Public Health.*

Steinemann A. 2017. Health and societal effects from exposure to fragranced consumer products. *Preventive Medicine Reports.*

Steinemann A. 2017. Ten questions concerning air fresheners and indoor built environments. *Building and Environment.*

Antibacterial Soaps

Ashurst JV, Nappe TM. 2019. Isopropanol toxicity. StatPearls.

Chen J, et al. 2018. Assessment of human exposure to triclocarban, triclosan and five parabens in U.S. indoor dust using dispersive solid phase extraction followed by liquid chromatography tandem mass spectrometry. *Journal of Hazardous Materials.*

Hipwell AE, et al. 2019. Exposure to non-persistent chemicals in consumer products and fecundability: a systematic review. *Human Reproductive Update.*

Jiang Y, et al. 2019. Prenatal exposure to benzophenones, parabens and triclosan and neurocognitive development at 2 years. *Environment International.*

Kim SA, et al. 2015. Bactericidal effects of triclosan in soap both in vitro and in vivo. *Journal of Antimicrobial Chemotherapy.*

Zhang H, et al. 2019. Integration of metabolomics and lipidomics reveals metabolic mechanisms of triclosan-induced toxicity in human hepatocytes. *Environmental Science & Technology.*

Antibiotic Ointments

Carson CF, Hammer KA, Riley TV. 2006. *Melaleuca alternifolia* (tea tree) oil: a review of antimicrobial and other medicinal properties. *Clinical Microbiology Reviews.*

Yap PS, et al. 2014. Essential oils, a new horizon in combating bacterial antibiotic resistance. *The Open Microbiology Journal.*

Bacteria

Al-Rawi A, Bahjat SA, Al-Allaf M. 2018. Novel natural disinfectants for contaminated cosmetic application tools. *International Journal of Medical Sciences.*

Christensen GJM, Brüggemann H. 2014. Bacterial skin commensals and their role as host guardians. *Beneficial Microbes.*

Song YM, et al. 2020. In vitro evaluation of the antibacterial properties of tea tree oil on planktonic and biofilm-forming *Streptococcus mutans.* *AAPS PharmSciTech.*

Bandages

Braun JM, Sathyanarayana S, Hauser R. 2013. Phthalate exposure and children's health. *Current Opinion in Pediatrics.*

Wallace MAG, Kormos TM, Pleil JD. 2016. Blood-borne biomarkers and bioindicators for linking exposure to health effects in environmental health science. *Journal of Toxicology and Environmental Health, Part B, Critical Reviews.*

Bath Bombs

Conklin DJ. 2016. Acute cardiopulmonary toxicity of inhaled aldehydes: role of TRPA1. *Annals of the New York Academy of Sciences.*

Cramer DW, et al. 2016. The association between talc use and ovarian cancer: a retrospective case-control study in two US states. *Epidemiology.*

Jurnak F. 2016. The pivotal role of aldehyde toxicity in autism spectrum disorder: the therapeutic potential of micronutrient supplementation. *Nutrition and Metabolic Insights*.

Penninkilampi R, Eslick GD. 2018. Perineal talc use and ovarian cancer: a systematic review and meta-analysis. *Epidemiology*.

Blush

Berger KP, et al. 2019. Personal care product use as a predictor of urinary concentrations of certain phthalates, parabens, and phenols in the HER-MOSA study. *Journal of Exposure Science & Environmental Epidemiology*.

Liu W, et al. 2019. Parabens exposure in early pregnancy and gestational diabetes mellitus. *Environment International*.

Nowak K, Jabłońska E, Ratajczak-Wrona W. 2019. Immunomodulatory effects of synthetic endocrine disrupting chemicals on the development and functions of human immune cells. *Environment International*.

Candles

Manigrasso M, et al. 2017. Temporal evolution of ultrafine particles and of alveolar deposited surface area from main indoor combustion and non-combustion sources in a model room. *Science of the Total Environment*.

Weber LP, et al. 2011. Role of carbon monoxide in impaired endothelial function mediated by acute second-hand tobacco, incense, and candle smoke exposures. *Environmental Toxicology and Pharmacology*.

Compact Powder

Al Awam KA, et al. 2019. The effect of cosmetic talc powder on health. *Indian Journal of Respiratory Care*.

Barros AI, et al. 2016. Effect of different precursors on generation of reference spectra for structural molecular background correction by solid sampling high-resolution continuum source graphite furnace atomic absorption spectrometry: determination of antimony in cosmetics. *Talanta*.

Fiume MM, et al. 2015. Safety assessment of ethanolamine and ethanolamine salts as used in cosmetics. *International Journal of Toxicology*.

Cosmetics

Berger KP, et al. 2019. Personal care product use as a predictor of urinary concentrations of certain phthalates, parabens, and phenols in the HER-MOSA study. *Journal of Exposure Science & Environmental Epidemiology*.

Calafat AM, et al. 2010. Urinary concentrations of four parabens in the U.S. population: NHANES 2005–2006. *Environmental Health Perspectives*.

Chen X, et al. 2018. Toxicity of cosmetic preservatives on human ocular surface and adnexal cells. *Experimental Eye Research*.

Jacob SL, et al. 2018. Cosmetics and cancer: adverse event reports submitted to the Food and Drug Administration. *JNCI Cancer Spectrum*.

Lim DS, et al. 2018. Non-cancer, cancer, and dermal sensitization risk assessment of heavy metals in cosmetics. *Journal of Toxicology and Environmental Health, Part A*.

Murat P, et al. 2019. Assessment of targeted non-intentionally added substances in cosmetics in contact with plastic packagings: analytical and toxicological aspects. *Food and Chemical Toxicology*.

Nguyen HL, Yiannias JA. 2019. Contact dermatitis to medications and skin products. *Clinical Reviews in Allergy & Immunology*.

Schultes L, et al. 2018. Per- and poly-fluoroalkyl substances and fluorine mass balance in cosmetic products from the Swedish market: implications for environmental emissions and human exposure. *Environmental Science: Processes & Impacts*.

Wang W, Kannan K. 2019. Quantitative identification of and exposure to synthetic phenolic antioxidants, including butylated hydroxytoluene, in urine. *Environment International*.

Deodorant

Linhart C, et al. 2017. Use of underarm cosmetic products in relation to risk of breast cancer: a case-control study. *EBioMedicine*.

Klotz K, et al. 2017. The health effects of aluminum exposure. *Deutsches Ärzteblatt International*.

Yoo J, et al. 2018. Potentiation of sodium metabisulfite toxicity by propylene glycol in both *in vitro* and *in vivo* systems. *Frontiers in Pharmacology*.

Zirwas MJ, Moennich J. 2008. Antiperspirant and deodorant allergy: diagnosis and management. *Journal of Clinical and Aesthetic Dermatology*.

Dust

Wei W, Mandin C, Ramalho O. 2018. Influence of indoor environmental factors on mass transfer parameters and concentrations of semi-volatile organic compounds. *Chemosphere*.

Exfoliants

Godoy V, et al. 2019. Physical-chemical characterization of microplastics present in some exfoliating products from Spain. *Marine Pollution Bulletin.*

Face Wash

Bernhoft RA. 2012. Mercury toxicity and treatment: a review of the literature. *Journal of Environmental and Public Health.*

Philippat C, et al. 2015. Exposure to select phthalates and phenols through use of personal care products among Californian adults and their children. *Environmental Research.*

Warshaw EM, et al. 2018. Contact dermatitis associated with skin cleansers: retrospective analysis of North American Contact Dermatitis Group data 2000–2014. *Dermatitis: Contact, Atopic, Occupational, Drug.*

Floss

Boronow KE, et al. 2019. Serum concentrations of PFASs and exposure-related behaviors in African American and non-Hispanic white women. *Journal of Exposure Science & Environmental Epidemiology.*

Fungi

Cadnum JL, et al. 2017. Effectiveness of disinfectants against *Candida auris* and other *Candida* species. *Infection Control & Hospital Epidemiology.*

Hair Conditioner

Fransway AF, et al. 2019. Paraben toxicology. *Dermatitis: Contact, Atopic, Occupational, Drug.*

Helm JS, et al. 2018. Measurement of endocrine disrupting and asthma-associated chemicals in hair products used by Black women. *Environmental Research.*

Sakhi AK, et al. 2017. Phthalate metabolites in Norwegian mothers and children: levels, diurnal variation and use of personal care products. *Science of the Total Environment.*

Hair Spray

Cogliano VJ, et al. 2011. Preventable exposures associated with human cancers. *Journal of the National Cancer Institute.*

Barrett JR. 2005. Chemical exposures: the ugly side of beauty products. *Environmental Health Perspectives.*

Infante PF, et al. 2009. Vinyl chloride propellant in hair spray and angiosarcoma of the liver among hairdressers and barbers: case reports. *International Journal of Occupational and Environmental Health.*

Musa OM, Tallon MA. 2013. Hair care polymers for styling and conditioning. In *Polymers for Personal Care and Cosmetics*, ed. A. Patil and MS Ferritto, 233–84. ACS Symposium Series, vol. 1148. Washington, D.C.: American Chemical Society.

Olsson A, Skogh T, Wingren G. 2001. Comorbidity and lifestyle, reproductive factors, and environmental exposures associated with rheumatoid arthritis. *Annals of the Rheumatic Diseases.*

Incense

Chen YC, Ho WC, Yu YH. 2017. Adolescent lung function associated with incense burning and other environmental exposures at home. *Indoor Air.*

Friborg JT, et al. 2008. Incense use and respiratory tract carcinomas: a prospective cohort study. *Cancer.*

Ndong Ba A, et al. 2019. Individual exposure level following indoor and outdoor air pollution exposure in Dakar (Senegal). *Environmental Pollution.*

Lip Balm

Gao P, et al. 2018. Bioaccessible trace metals in lip cosmetics and their health risks to female consumers. *Environmental Pollution.*

Kaličanin B, Velimirović D. 2016. A study of the possible harmful effects of cosmetic beauty products on human health. *Biological Trace Element Research.*

Lipstick

Hsieh CJ, et al. 2019. Personal care products use and phthalate exposure levels among pregnant women. *Science of the Total Environment.*

Kazi TG, et al. 2019. A rapid ultrasonic energy assisted preconcentration method for simultaneous extraction of lead and cadmium in various cosmetic brands using deep eutectic solvent: a multivariate study. *Ultrasonics Sonochemistry.*

Monnot AD, et al. 2015. An exposure and health risk assessment of lead (Pb) in lipstick. *Food and Chemical Toxicology.*

Lotion

Drechsel DA, et al. 2018. Skin sensitization induction potential from daily exposure to fragrances in personal care products. *Dermatitis: Contact, Atopic, Occupational, Drug.*

Engel SM, et al. 2018. Prenatal phthalates, maternal thyroid function, and risk of attention-deficit hyperactivity disorder in the Norwegian Mother and Child Cohort. *Environmental Health Perspectives.*

Menstrual Products

Branch F, et al. 2015. Vaginal douching and racial/ethnic disparities in phthalates exposures among reproductive-aged women: National Health and Nutrition Examination Survey 2001–2004. *Environmental Health.*

Dudley S, et al. 2022. Tampon safety. National Center for Health Research website.

Gelbke HP, et al. 2009. A review of health effects of carbon disulfide in viscose industry and a proposal for an occupational exposure limit. *Critical Reviews in Toxicology*.

McDermott C, Sheridan M. 2015. Staphylococcal toxic shock syndrome caused by tampon use. *Case Reports in Critical Care*.

Park CJ, et al. 2019. Sanitary pads and diapers contain higher phthalate contents than those in common commercial plastic products. *Reproductive Toxicology*.

Sieja K, von Mach-Szczypinski J, von Mach-Szczypinski J. 2018. Health effect of chronic exposure to carbon disulfide (C2) on women employed in viscose industry. *Medycyna Pracy*.

Mouthwash

Bashash M, et al. 2017. Prenatal fluoride exposure and cognitive outcomes in children at 4 and 6–12 years of age in Mexico. *Environmental Health Perspectives*.

Choi AL, et al. 2012. Developmental fluoride neurotoxicity: a systematic review and meta-analysis. *Environmental Health Perspectives*.

Grandjean P, Landrigan PJ. 2014. Neurobehavioural effects of developmental toxicity. *The Lancet Neurology*.

Kolikonda MK, et al. 2014. A case of mouthwash as a source of ethanol poisoning: is there a need to limit alcohol content of mouthwash? *The Primary Care Companion for CNS Disorders*.

Nakamoto T, Rawls HR. 2018. Fluoride exposure in early life as the possible root cause of disease in later life. *Journal of Clinical Pediatric Dentistry*.

Peckham S, Awofeso N. 2014. Water fluoridation: a critical review of the physiological effects of ingested fluoride as a public health intervention. *The Scientific World Journal*.

Salvatori C, et al. 2017. A comparative study of antibacterial and anti-inflammatory effects of mouthrinse containing tea tree oil. *ORAL & Implantology*.

Sauerheber R. 2013. Physiologic conditions affect toxicity of ingested industrial fluoride. *Journal of Environmental and Public Health*.

Somaraj V, et al. 2017. Effect of herbal and fluoride mouth rinses on *Streptococcus mutans* and dental caries among 12–15-year-old school children: a randomized controlled trial. *International Journal of Dentistry*.

Nail Polish

Tanaka A, Leung PS, Gershwin ME. 2018. Environmental basis of primary biliary cholangitis. *Experimental Biology and Medicine*.

Young AS, et al. 2018. Phthalate and organophosphate plasticizers in nail polish: evaluation of labels and ingredients. *Environmental Science & Technology*.

Nail Polish Remover

Butt CM, et al. 2016. Regional comparison of organophosphate flame retardant (PFR) urinary metabolites and tetrabromobenzoic acid (TBBA) in mother-toddler pairs from California and New Jersey. *Environment International*.

Mendelsohn E, et al. 2016. Nail polish as a source of exposure to triphenyl phosphate. *Environment International*.

Vitale CM, Gutovitz S. 2019. Aromatic (benzene, toluene) toxicity. StatPearls.

Perfume

Al-Saleh I, Elkhatib R. 2016. Screening of phthalate esters in 47 branded perfumes. *Environmental Science and Pollution Research*.

Silva-Néto RP, et al. 2017. May headache triggered by odors be regarded as a differentiating factor between migraine and other primary headaches? *Cephalalgia*.

Sowndhararajan K, Kim S. 2016. Influence of fragrances on human psychophysiological activity: with special reference to human electroencephalographic response. *Scientia Pharmaceutica*.

Personal Care Products

Chen SC, et al. 2010. Endocrine disruptor, dioxin (TCDD)-induced mitochondrial dysfunction and apoptosis in human trophoblast-like JAR cells. *Molecular Human Reproduction*.

Rier S, Foster WG. 2002. Environmental dioxins and endometriosis. *Toxicological Sciences*.

Wendee N. 2014. A question for women's health: chemicals in feminine hygiene products and personal lubricants. *Environmental Health Perspectives*.

Shampoo

Craciunescu CN, Wu R, Zeisel SH. 2006. Diethanolamine alters neurogenesis and induces apoptosis in fetal mouse hippocampus. *The FASEB Journal*.

Fisher M, et al. 2017. Paraben concentrations in maternal urine and breast milk and its association with personal care product use. *Environmental Science & Technology*.

Helm JS, et al. 2018. Measurement of endocrine disrupting and asthma-associated chemicals in hair products used by Black women. *Environmental Research*.

Panchal SR, Verma RJ. 2013. Spermatotoxic effect of diethanolamine: an *in vitro* study. *Asian Pacific Journal of Reproduction*.

Philippat C, et al. 2015. Exposure to select phthalates and phenols through use of personal care products among Californian adults and their children. *Environmental Research*.

Shaving Cream
Borowska S, Brzóska MM. 2018. Metals in cosmetics: implications for human health. *Metal Allergy: From Dermatitis to Implant and Device Failure*.

Harley KG, et al. 2016. Reducing phthalate, paraben, and phenol exposure from personal care products in adolescent girls: findings from the HERMOSA Intervention Study. *Environmental Health Perspectives*.

Shower Curtains
Hannon PR, Flaws JA. 2015. The effects of phthalates on the ovary. *Frontiers in Endocrinology*.

Latorre I, et al. 2012. PVC biodeterioration and DEHP leaching by DEHP-degrading bacteria. *International Biodeterioration & Biodegradation*.

Lester S, Schade M, Weigand C. 2008. *Volatile Vinyl: The New Shower Curtain's Chemical Smell*. Falls Church, Va.: Center for Health, Environment and Justice.

Showerheads
Chang CW, Chou FC. 2011. Methodologies for quantifying culturable, viable, and total *Legionella pneumophila* in indoor air. *Indoor Air*.

Gebert MJ, et al. 2018. Ecological analyses of mycobacteria in showerhead biofilms and their relevance to human health. *mBio*.

Higa F, et al. 2012. *Legionella pneumophila* contamination in a steam towel warmer in a hospital setting. *The Journal of Hospital Infection*.

Soap
Sakhi AK, et al. 2017. Phthalate metabolites in Norwegian mothers and children: levels, diurnal variation and use of personal care products. *Science of the Total Environment*.

Sunscreen
DiNardo JC, Downs CA. 2018. Dermatological and environmental toxicological impact of the sunscreen ingredient oxybenzone/benzophenone-3. *Journal of Cosmetic Dermatology*.

Ghazipura M, et al. 2017. Exposure to benzophenone-3 and reproductive toxicity: a systematic review of human and animal studies. *Reproductive Toxicology*.

Ruszkiewicz JA, et al. 2017. Neurotoxic effect of active ingredients in sunscreen products, a contemporary review. *Toxicology Reports*.

Schneider SL, Lim HW. 2019. Review of environmental effects of oxybenzone and other sunscreen active ingredients. *Journal of the American Academy of Dermatology*.

Talcum Powder
Berge W, et al. 2018. Genital use of talc and risk of ovarian cancer: a meta-analysis. *European Journal of Cancer Prevention*.

Teeth Whitening
Tadros J, Patel F, Keenan K. 2019. Degradation of proteins extracted from teeth by hydrogen peroxide. *The FASEB Journal*.

Valkenburg, C, et al. 2019. The efficacy of baking soda dentifrice in controlling plaque and gingivitis: a systematic review. *International Journal of Dental Hygiene*.

Toilet
Barker J, Jones MV. 2005. The potential spread of infection caused by aerosol contamination of surfaces after flushing a domestic toilet. *Journal of Applied Microbiology*.

Johnson DL, et al. 2013. Lifting the lid on toilet plume aerosol: a literature review with suggestions for future research. *American Journal of Infection Control*.

Mughal BB, Fini JB, Demeneix BA. 2018. Thyroid-disrupting chemicals and brain development: an update. *Endocrine Connections*.

Toilet Paper
Bethea TN, et al. 2019. Correlates of exposure to phenols, parabens, and triclocarban in the Study of Environment, Lifestyle and Fibroids. *Journal of Exposure Science & Environmental Epidemiology*.

Liao C, Kannan K. 2011. Widespread occurrence of bisphenol A in paper and paper products: implications for human exposure. *Environmental Science & Technology*.

Wang Z, et al. 2019. Bisphenol A and pubertal height growth in school-aged children. *Journal of Exposure Science & Environmental Epidemiology*.

Toothbrush
Bhoil R, Bhoil R. 2016. Toothbrush contamination: often neglected health hazard. *Journal of Family Medicine and Primary Care*.

Chlubek D, Sikora M. 2020. Fluoride and pineal gland. *Applied Sciences*.

Han J, et al. 2017. Nylon bristles and elastomers retain centigram levels of triclosan and other chemicals from toothpastes: accumulation and uncontrolled release. *Environmental Science & Technology*.

Thamke MV, et al. 2018. Comparison of bacterial contamination and antibacterial efficacy in bristles of charcoal toothbrushes versus noncharcoal toothbrushes: a microbiological study. *Contemporary Clinical Dentistry*.

Van Leeuwen MPC, et al. 2018. Toothbrush wear in relation to toothbrushing effectiveness. *International Journal of Dental Hygiene*.

Weatherly LM, Gosse JA. 2017. Triclosan exposure, transformation, and human health effects. *Journal of Toxicology and Environmental Health, Part B*.

Toothpaste

Anderson AG, et al. 2016. Microplastics in personal care products: exploring perceptions of environmentalists, beauticians and students. *Marine Pollution Bulletin*.

Basch CH, Kernan WD. 2016. Ingredients in children's fluoridated toothpaste: a literature review. *Global Journal of Health Science*.

Dagli N, et al. 2015. Essential oils, their therapeutic properties, and implication in dentistry: a review. *Journal of International Society of Preventive & Community Dentistry*.

Hans VM, et al. 2016. Antimicrobial efficacy of various essential oils at varying concentrations against periopathogen *Porphyromonas gingivalis*. *Journal of Clinical and Diagnostic Research: JCDR*.

Hara AT, Turssi CP. 2017. Baking soda as an abrasive in toothpastes: mechanism of action and safety and effectiveness considerations. *The Journal of the American Dental Association*.

Kumar V, et al. 2018. Fluoride, thyroid hormone derangements and its correlation with tooth eruption pattern among the pediatric population from endemic and non-endemic fluorosis areas. *The Journal of Contemporary Dental Practice*.

Malin AJ, et al. 2018. Fluoride exposure and thyroid function among adults living in Canada: effect modification by iodine status. *Environment International*.

Malin AJ, et al. 2019. Fluoride exposure and kidney and liver function among adolescents in the United States: NHANES, 2013–2016. *Environment International*.

Peedikayil FC, Sreenivasan P, Narayanan A. 2015. Effect of coconut oil in plaque related gingivitis: a preliminary report. *Nigerian Medical Journal*.

Pycke BFG, et al. 2014. Human fetal exposure to triclosan and triclocarban in an urban population from Brooklyn, New York. *Environmental Science & Technology*.

Song YM, et al. 2020. In vitro evaluation of the antibacterial properties of tea tree oil on planktonic and biofilm-forming *Streptococcus mutans*. *AAPS PharmSciTech*.

Thornton-Evans G, et al. 2019. Use of toothpaste and toothbrushing patterns among children and adolescents— United States, 2013–2016. *Morbidity and Mortality Weekly Report*.

Tsai ML, et al. 2013. Chemical composition and biological properties of essential oils of two mint species. *Tropical Journal of Pharmaceutical Research*.

Ullah R, Zafar MS, Shahani N. 2017. Potential fluoride toxicity from oral medicaments: a review. *Iranian Journal of Basic Medical Sciences*.

Varma SR, et al. 2018. The antiplaque efficacy of two herbal-based toothpastes: a clinical intervention. *Journal of International Society of Preventive & Community Dentistry*.

Triclosan

Calafat AM, et al. 2008. Urinary concentrations of triclosan in the U.S. population: 2003–2004. *Environmental Health Perspectives*.

Halden RU, et al. 2017. The Florence statement on triclosan and triclocarban. *Environmental Health Perspectives*.

CHAPTER FOUR: BEDROOM

Bed Frames

Dezest M, et al. 2017. Oxidative damage and impairment of protein quality control systems in keratinocytes exposed to a volatile organic compounds cocktail. *Scientific Reports*.

Ho DX, et al. 2011. Emission rates of volatile organic compounds released from newly produced household furniture products using a large-scale chamber testing method. *The Scientific World Journal*.

Jones M, et al. 2018. Thermal degradation and fire properties of fungal mycelium and mycelium-biomass composite materials. *Scientific Reports*.

Kim KW, et al. 2010. Formaldehyde and TVOC emission behaviors according to finishing treatment with surface materials using 20 L chamber and FLEC. *Journal of Hazardous Materials*.

Liu R, et al. 2018. Characterization of odors of wood by gas chromatography-olfactometry with removal of extractives as attempt to control indoor air quality. *Molecules*.

Mendell MJ. 2007. Indoor residential chemical emissions as risk factors for respiratory and allergic effects in children: a review. *Indoor Air*.

Closets

Avagyan R, et al. 2015. Benzothiazole, benzotriazole, and their derivatives in clothing textiles—potential source of environmental pollutants and human exposure. *Environmental Science and Pollution Research.*

Iadaresta F, et al. 2018. Chemicals from textiles to skin: an in vitro permeation study of benzothiazole. *Environmental Science and Pollution Research.*

Rovira J, et al. 2015. Human exposure to trace elements through the skin by direct contact with clothing: risk assessment. *Environmental Research.*

Dust

Fessler MB, et al. 2017. House dust endotoxin and peripheral leukocyte counts: results from two large epidemiologic studies. *Environmental Health Perspectives.*

Kassotis CD, Hoffman K, Stapleton HM. 2017. Characterization of adipogenic activity of house dust extracts and semi-volatile indoor contaminants in 3T3-L1 cells. *Environmental Science & Technology.*

Kassotis CD, et al. 2019. Thyroid receptor antagonism as a contributory mechanism for adipogenesis induced by environmental mixtures in 3T3-L1 cells. *Science of the Total Environment.*

Salo, PM, Cohn RD, Zeldin DC. 2018. Bedroom allergen exposure beyond house dust mites. *Current Allergy and Asthma Reports.*

Mattresses

Gaire S, Scharf ME, Gondhalekar AD. 2019. Toxicity and neurophysiological impacts of plant essential oil components on bed bugs (Cimicidae: Hemiptera). *Scientific Reports.*

Kwon JW, et al. 2018. Exposure to volatile organic compounds and airway inflammation. *Environmental Health.*

Lounis M, et al. 2019. Fireproofing of domestic upholstered furniture: migration of flame retardants and potential risks. *Journal of Hazardous Materials.*

Makey CM, et al. 2016. Polybrominated diphenyl ether exposure and thyroid function tests in North American adults. *Environmental Health Perspectives.*

Portnoy J, et al. 2013. Environmental assessment and exposure control of dust mites: a practice parameter. *Annals of Allergy, Asthma & Immunology.*

Schupp T. 2018. Derivation of indoor air guidance values for volatile organic compounds (VOC) emitted from polyurethane flexible foam: VOC with repeated dose toxicity data. *EXCLI Journal.*

Mothballs

Dubey D, et al. 2014. Para-dichlorobenzene toxicity—a review of potential neurotoxic manifestations. *Therapeutic Advancements in Neurological Disorders.*

Sudakin DL, Stone DL, Power L. 2011. Naphthalene mothballs: emerging and recurring issues and their relevance to environmental health. *Current Topics in Toxicology.*

Volney G, et al. 2018. Naphthalene toxicity: methemoglobinemia and acute intravascular hemolysis. *Cureus.*

Pillows

Baxi SN, et al. 2016. Exposure and health effects of fungi on humans. *The Journal of Allergy and Clinical Immunology: In Practice.*

Woodcock AA, et al. 2006. Fungal contamination of bedding. *Allergy.*

Xu W, et al.. 2018. Emission of sulfur dioxide from polyurethane foam and respiratory health effects. *Environmental Pollution.*

Sheets and Mattress Pads

Dezest M, et al. 2017. Oxidative damage and impairment of protein quality control systems in keratinocytes exposed to a volatile organic compounds cocktail. *Scientific Reports.*

Hauptmann M, et al. 2003. Mortality from lymphohematopoietic malignancies among workers in formaldehyde industries. *Journal of the National Cancer Institute.*

Rovira J, Domingo JL. 2019. Human health risks due to exposure to inorganic and organic chemicals from textiles: a review. *Environmental Research.*

Sak ZHA, et al. 2018. Respiratory symptoms and pulmonary functions before and after pesticide application in cotton farming. *Annals of Agricultural and Environmental Medicine.*

CHAPTER FIVE: LIVING ROOM

Carpet

Katsoyiannis A, Leva P, Kotzias D. 2008. VOC and carbonyl emissions from carpets: a comparative study using four types of environmental chambers. *Journal of Hazardous Materials.*

Kim M, et al. 2015. Compositional effects on leaching of stain-guarded (perfluoroalkyl and polyfluoroalkyl substance-treated) carpet in landfill leachate. *Environmental Science & Technology.*

Lucattini L, et al. 2018. A review of semi-volatile organic compounds (SVOCs) in the indoor environment: occurrence in consumer products, indoor air and dust. *Chemosphere.*

Yang C, et al. 2018. Early-life exposure to endocrine disrupting chemicals associates with childhood obesity. *Annals of Pediatric Endocrinology & Metabolism.*

Curtains

Hartwig A. 2013. Cadmium and cancer. *Cadmium: From Toxicity to Essentiality. Metal Ions in Life Sciences, Vol. 11.*

Fireplace

Francisco PW, Gordon JR, Rose B. 2010. Measured concentrations of combustion gases from the use of unvented gas fireplaces. *Indoor Air.*

Hosgood HD III, et al. 2010. In-home coal and wood use and lung cancer risk: a pooled analysis of the International Lung Cancer Consortium. *Environmental Health Perspectives.*

White AJ, Sandler DP. 2017. Indoor wood-burning stove and fireplace use and breast cancer in a prospective cohort study. *Environmental Health Perspectives.*

Leather Furniture

Fleisch AF, et al. 2017. Early-life exposure to perfluoroalkyl substances and childhood metabolic function. *Environmental Health Perspectives.*

Kotthoff M, et al. 2015. Perfluoroalkyl and polyfluoroalkyl substances in consumer products. *Environmental Science and Pollution Research.*

Plants

Teiri H, Pourzamzni H, Hajizadeh Y. 2018. Phytoremediation of formaldehyde from indoor environment by ornamental plants: an approach to promote occupants health. *International Journal of Preventive Medicine.*

Wolverton BC. 2019. NASA plant research offers a breath of fresh air. NASA Spinoff website.

Television Screens

Grellier J, Ravazzani P, Cardis E. 2014. Potential health impacts of residential exposures to extremely low frequency magnetic fields in Europe. *Environment International.*

Huss A, et al. 2018. Occupational extremely low frequency magnetic fields (ELF-MF) exposure and hematolymphopoietic cancers— Swiss National Cohort analysis and updated meta-analysis. *Environmental Research.*

Sun ZC, et al. 2016. Extremely low frequency electromagnetic fields facilitate vesicle endocytosis by increasing presynaptic calcium channel expression at a central synapse. *Scientific Reports.*

Upholstery

Butt CM, et al. 2014. Metabolites of organophosphate flame retardants and 2-ethylhexyl tetrabromobenzoate in urine from paired mothers and toddlers. *Environmental Science & Technology.*

Hammel SC, et al. 2017. Associations between flame retardant applications in furniture foam, house dust levels, and residents' serum levels. *Environment International.*

Harris MH, et al. 2017. Predictors of per- and polyfluoroalkyl substance (PFAS) plasma concentrations in 6–10 year old American children. *Environmental Science & Technology.*

Hoffman K, et al. 2015. Monitoring indoor exposure to organophosphate flame retardants: hand wipes and house dust. *Environmental Health Perspectives.*

McGrath TJ, et al. 2018. Concentrations of legacy and novel brominated flame retardants in indoor dust in Melbourne, Australia: an assessment of human exposure. *Environment International.*

Stapleton HM, et al. 2012. Novel and high volume use flame retardants in US couches reflective of the 2005 PentaBDE phase out. *Environmental Science & Technology.*

Tong RP, et al. 2018. [Source analysis and environmental health risk assessment of VOCs in furniture manufacturing.] *Huan Jing ke Xue.* Article in Chinese.

Winkens K, et al. 2017. Early life exposure to per- and polyfluoroalkyl substances (PFASs): a critical review. *Emerging Contaminants.*

Yao Y, et al. 2018. Per- and polyfluoroalkyl substances (PFASs) in indoor air and dust from homes and various microenvironments in China: implications for human exposure. *Environmental Science & Technology.*

Wood Furniture

Ho DX, et al. 2011. Emission rates of volatile organic compounds released from newly produced household furniture products using a large-scale chamber testing method. *Scientific World Journal.*

Schecter A, et al. 2003. Polybrominated diphenyl ethers (PBDEs) in U.S. mothers' milk. *Environmental Health Perspectives.*

Tormoehlen LM, Tekulve KJ, Nañagas KA. 2014. Hydrocarbon toxicity: a review. *Clinical Toxicology.*

CHAPTER SIX: LAUNDRY ROOM

Bleach

Leri AC, Anthony LN. 2013. Formation of organochlorine by-products in bleached laundry. *Chemosphere.*

Dryer Lint

Saini A, et al. 2016. From clothing to laundry water: investigating the fate of phthalates, brominated flame retardants, and organophosphate esters. *Environmental Science & Technology.*

Stapleton HM, et al. 2005. Polybrominated diphenyl ethers in house dust and clothes dryer lint. *Environmental Science & Technology.*

Steinemann A, et al. 2013. Chemical emissions from residential dryer vents during use of fragranced laundry products. *Air Quality, Atmosphere & Health.*

Sun J, et al. 2018. Emissions of selected brominated flame retardants from consumer materials: the effects of content, temperature, and timescale. *Environmental Science and Pollution Research.*

Dryer Sheets

Caress SM, Steinemann AC. 2009. Prevalence of fragrance sensitivity in the American population. *Journal of Environmental Health.*

Dodson RE, et al. 2012. Endocrine disruptors and asthma-associated chemicals in consumer products. *Environmental Health Perspectives.*

Potera C. 2011. Indoor air quality: scented products emit a bouquet of VOCs. *Environmental Health Perspectives.*

Steinemann AC. 2016. Fragranced consumer products: exposures and effects from emissions. *Air Quality, Atmosphere & Health.*

Dryer Vents

Goodman NB, et al. 2019. Emissions from dryer vents during use of fragranced and fragrance-free laundry products. *Air Quality, Atmosphere & Health.*

Kessler R. 2011. Dryer vents: an overlooked source of pollution? *Environmental Health Perspectives.*

Steinemann AC, et al. 2013. Chemical emissions from residential dryer vents during use of fragranced laundry products. *Air Quality, Atmosphere & Health.*

Fabric Softener

Anderson RC, Anderson JH. 2000. Respiratory toxicity of fabric softener emissions. *Journal of Toxicology and Environmental Health, Part A.*

Laundry Detergent

Bonney AG, Mazor S, Goldman RD. 2013. Laundry detergent capsules and pediatric poisoning. *Canadian Family Physician.*

Cheng M, et al. 2016. Factors controlling volatile organic compounds in dwellings in Melbourne, Australia. *Indoor Air.*

Davis MG, et al. 2016. Pediatric exposures to laundry and dishwasher detergents in the United States: 2013–2014. *Pediatrics.*

Jardak K, Drogui P, Daghrir R. 2016. Surfactants in aquatic and terrestrial environment: occurrence, behavior, and treatment processes. *Environmental Science and Pollution Research.*

Mesnage R, Antoniou MN. 2018. Ignoring adjuvant toxicity falsifies the safety profile of commercial pesticides. *Frontiers in Public Health.*

Seweryn A. 2018. Interactions between surfactants and the skin—theory and practice. *Advances in Colloid and Interface Science.*

Sjogren PP, Skarda DE, Park AH. 2017. Upper aerodigestive injuries from detergent ingestion in children. *The Laryngoscope.*

Wang M, et al. 2018. Laundry detergents and detergent residue after rinsing directly disrupt tight junction barrier integrity in human bronchial epithelial cells. *The Journal of Allergy and Clinical Immunology.*

Stain Remover

Hong S, et al. 2014. Association between exposure to antimicrobial household products and allergic symptoms. *Environmental Health and Toxicology.*

Wang G, et al. 2017. Autoimmune potential of perchloroethylene: role of lipid-derived aldehydes. *Toxicology and Applied Pharmacology.*

Static Spray

Robinson AJ, et al. 2017. Granular parakeratosis induced by benzalkonium chloride exposure from laundry rinse aids. *Australasian Journal of Dermatology.*

CHAPTER SEVEN: KIDS' ROOMS

Baby Monitors

Moon JH. Health effects of electromagnetic fields on children. 2020. *Clinical and Experimental Pediatrics.*

Sage C, Burgio E. 2018. Electromagnetic fields, pulsed radiofrequency radiation, and epigenetics: how wireless technologies may affect childhood development. *Child Development.*

Baby Wipes

Celeiro M, et al. 2015. Pressurized liquid extraction-gas chromatography-mass spectrometry analysis of fragrance allergens, musks, phthalates and preservatives in baby wipes. *Journal of Chromatography A.*

Gosens I, et al. 2014. Aggregate exposure approaches for parabens in personal care products: a case assessment for children between 0 and 3 years old. *Journal of Exposure Science & Environmental Epidemiology.*

Halla N, et al. 2018. Cosmetics preservation: a review on present strategies. *Molecules.*

Jang HJ, Shin CY, Kim KB. 2015. Safety evaluation of polyethylene glycol (PEG) compounds for cosmetic use. *Toxicological Research.*

Neu L, et al. 2018. Ugly ducklings—the dark side of plastic materials in contact with potable water. *npj Biofilms and Microbiomes.*

Bassinet

Bornehag CG, et al. 2018. Association of prenatal phthalate exposure with language development in early childhood. *JAMA Pediatrics.*

Stapleton HM, et al. 2011. Identification of flame retardants in polyurethane foam collected from baby products. *Environmental Science & Technology.*

Bedding (Sheets/Blankets)

Alvarado-Cruz I, et al. 2018. Environmental epigenetic changes, as risk factors for the development of diseases in children: a systematic review. *Annals of Global Health.*

Bakian AV, VanDerslice JA. 2019. Pesticides and autism. *The British Medical Journal.*

Boor BE, et al. 2015. Identification of phthalate and alternative plasticizers, flame retardants, and unreacted isocyanates in infant crib mattress covers and foam. *Environmental Science & Technology Letters.*

Sarwar M, Lee A. 2016. Indoor risks of pesticide uses are significantly linked to hazards of the family members. *Cogent Medicine.*

von Ehrenstein OS, et al. 2019. Prenatal and infant exposure to ambient pesticides and autism spectrum disorder in children: population based case-control study. *The British Medical Journal.*

Bottles and Pacifiers

Stacy SL, et al. 2016. Patterns, variability, and predictors of urinary bisphenol A concentrations during childhood. *Environmental Science & Technology.*

Carpeting

Zhou J, Mainelis G, Weisel CP. 2019. Pyrethroid levels in toddlers' breathing zone following a simulated indoor pesticide spray. *Journal of Exposure Science & Environmental Epidemiology.*

Clothes

Iadaresta F, et al. 2018. Chemicals from textiles to skin: an in vitro permeation study of benzothiazole. *Environmental Science and Pollution Research.*

Liu W, Xue J, Kannan K. 2017. Occurrence of and exposure to benzothiazoles and benzotriazoles from textiles and infant clothing. *Science of the Total Environment.*

Rovira J, et al. 2015. Human exposure to trace elements through the skin by direct contact with clothing: risk assessment. *Environmental Research.*

Cosmetic Products for Babies and Kids

Agier L, et al. 2019. Early-life exposome and lung function in children in Europe: an analysis of data from the longitudinal, population-based HELIX cohort. *The Lancet Planetary Health.*

Ginsberg G, Ginsberg J, Foos B. 2016. Approaches to children's exposure assessment: case study with diethyl-hexylphthalate (DEHP). *International Journal of Environmental Research and Public Health.*

Low KY, Wallace M. 2019. Prevalence of potential contact allergens in baby cosmetic products. *Clinical and Experimental Dermatology.*

Zhou J, et al. 2017. Estimating infants' and toddlers' inhalation exposure to fragrance ingredients in baby personal care products. *International Journal of Occupational and Environmental Health.*

Costumes

Eskenazi B, et al. 2013. *In utero* and childhood polybrominated diphenyl ether (PBDE) exposures and neurodevelopment in the CHAMACOS study. *Environmental Health Perspectives.*

Soubry A, et al. 2017. Human exposure to flame-retardants is associated with aberrant DNA methylation at imprinted genes in sperm. *Environmental Epigenetics.*

Crib Mattresses and Mattress Covers

Boor BE, et al. 2014. Infant exposure to emissions of volatile organic compounds from crib mattresses. *Environmental Science and Technology.*

Liang Y, Xu Y. 2014. Emission of phthalates and phthalate alternatives from vinyl flooring and crib mattress covers: the influence of temperature. *Environmental Science & Technology.*

Cribs

Butt CM, et al. 2016. Regional comparison of organophosphate flame retardant (PFR) urinary metabolites and tetrabromobenzoic acid (TBBA) in mother-toddler pairs from California and New Jersey. *Environment International.*

Curtains

Kim JH, Seok K. 2019. Combined assessment of preschool childrens' exposure to substances in household products. *International Journal of Environmental Research and Public Health.*

Diapers

Alberta L, Sweeney SM, Wiss K. 2005. Diaper dye dermatitis. *Pediatrics.*

Bender JK, Faergemann J, Sköld M. 2017. Skin health connected to the use of absorbent hygiene products: a review. *Dermatology and Therapy.*

Lagadic L, et al. 2017. Tributyltin: advancing the science on assessing endocrine disruption with an unconventional endocrine-disrupting compound. *Reviews of Environmental Contamination and Toxicology.*

Park CJ, et al. 2019. Sanitary pads and diapers contain higher phthalate contents than those in common commercial plastic products. *Reproductive Toxicology.*

Umachitra G, Bhaarathidhurai. 2012. Disposable baby diaper—a threat to the health and environment. *Journal of Environmental Science & Engineering.*

Dust

Butt CM, et al. 2014. Metabolites of organophosphate flame retardants and 2-ethylhexyl tetrabromobenzoate in urine from paired mothers and toddlers. *Environmental Science & Technology.*

Coakley JD, et al. 2013. Concentrations of polybrominated diphenyl ethers in matched samples of indoor dust and breast milk in New Zealand. *Environment International.*

Glenn L. 2015. Pick your poison: what's new in poison control for the preschooler. *Journal of Pediatric Nursing.*

Electronics

Bonafide CP, Jamison DT, Foglia EE. 2017. The emerging market of smartphone-integrated infant physiologic monitors. *JAMA.*

Morgan LL, Kesari S, Davis DL. 2014. Why children absorb more microwave radiation than adults: the consequences. *Journal of Microscopy and Ultrastructure.*

Sage C, Carpenter DO. 2009. Public health implications of wireless technologies. *Pathophysiology.*

Mattresses

Chevrier J, et al. 2010. Polybrominated diphenyl ether (PBDE) flame retardants and thyroid hormone during pregnancy. *Environmental Health Perspectives.*

Cowell WJ, et al. 2018. Temporal trends and developmental patterns of plasma polybrominated diphenyl ether concentrations over a 15-year period between 1998 and 2013. *Journal of Exposure Science & Environmental Epidemiology.*

Cowell WJ, et al. 2019. Pre- and postnatal polybrominated diphenyl ether concentrations in relation to thyroid parameters measured during early childhood. *Thyroid.*

Morello-Frosch R, et al. 2016. Environmental chemicals in an urban population of pregnant women and their newborns from San Francisco. *Environmental Science & Technology.*

Yu M, et al. 2016. Crib mattress investigation: a quality improvement study to assess mattress cover permeability and bacterial growth in crib mattresses. *American Journal of Infection Control.*

Stuffed Animals

Stapleton HM, et al. 2011. Identification of flame retardants in polyurethane foam collected from baby products. *Environmental Science & Technology.*

Tents

Gomes G, et al. 2016. Characterizing flame retardant applications and potential human exposure in backpacking tents. *Environmental Science & Technology.*

Keller AS, et al. 2014. Flame retardant applications in camping tents and potential exposure. *Environmental Science & Technology Letters.*

Toys

Ashworth, MJ, et al. 2018. Analysis and assessment of exposure to selected phthalates found in children's toys in Christchurch, New Zealand. *International Journal of Environmental Research and Public Health.*

Becker M, Edwards S, Massey RI. 2010. Toxic chemicals in toys and children's products: limitations of current responses and recommendations for government and industry. *Environmental Science & Technology.*

Hoffman K, et al. 2017. Toddler's behavior and its impacts on exposure to polybrominated diphenyl ethers. *Journal of Exposure Science & Environmental Epidemiology.*

Kadawathagedara M, de Lauzon-Guillain B, Botton J. 2018. Environmental contaminants and child's growth. *Journal of Developmental Origins of Health and Disease.*

Lin LY, et al. 2018. Childhood exposure to phthalates and pulmonary function. *Science of the Total Environment.*

Negev M, et al. 2018. Concentrations of trace metals, phthalates, bisphenol A and flame-retardants in toys and other children's products in Israel. *Chemosphere.*

Pell T, et al. 2017. Parental concern about environmental chemical exposures and children's urinary concentrations of phthalates and phenols. *The Journal of Pediatrics.*

CHAPTER EIGHT: HOME OFFICE

Acrylic Paints

Bauer P, Buettner A. 2018. Characterization of odorous and potentially harmful substances in artists' acrylic paint. *Frontiers in Public Health.*

Air

Du L, et al. 2015. Air exchange rates and migration of VOCs in basements and residences. *Indoor Air.*

Ammonia

Kant S, et al. 2019. Ethanol sensitizes skeletal muscle to ammonia-induced molecular perturbations. *Journal of Biological Chemistry.*

Chairs

Betts KS. 2015. Hand-me-down hazard: flame retardants in discarded foam products. *Environmental Health Perspectives.*

Schupp T. 2018. Derivation of indoor air guidance values for volatile organic compounds (VOC) emitted from polyurethane flexible foam: VOC with repeated dose toxicity data. *EXCLI Journal*.

Electromagnetic Fields (EMFs)

Falcioni L, et al. 2018. Report of final results regarding brain and heart tumors in Sprague-Dawley rats exposed from prenatal life until natural death to mobile phone radiofrequency field representative of a 1.8 GHz GSM base station environmental emission. *Environmental Research*.

Feldman Y, Ben-Ishai P. 2017. Potential risks to human health originating from future sub-MM communication systems. Transcript of a lecture by Paul Ben-Ishai at the January 2017 Israel Institute for Advanced Studies Conference at Hebrew University, Jerusalem, Israel.

Foster KR, Tell RA. 2013. Radiofrequency energy exposure from the Trilliant smart meter. *Health Physics*.

Hao YH, Zhao L, Peng RY. 2015. Effects of microwave radiation on brain energy metabolism and related mechanisms. *Military Medical Research*.

Hardell L. 2017. World Health Organization, radiofrequency radiation and health—a hard nut to crack (review). *International Journal of Oncology*.

Hardell L, Carlberg M. 2019. Comments on the US National Toxicology Program technical reports on toxicology and carcinogenesis study in rats exposed to whole-body radiofrequency radiation at 900 MHz and in mice exposed to whole-body radiofrequency radiation at 1,900 MHz. *International Journal of Oncology*.

Kamali K, et al. 2017. Effects of electromagnetic waves emitted from 3G+wi-fi modems on human semen analysis. *Urologia*.

Kelley E, et al. 2015. International appeal: scientists call for protection from non-ionizing electromagnetic field exposure. *European Journal of Oncology*.

Kesari KK, Agarwal A, Henkel R. 2018. Radiations and male fertility. *Reproductive Biology and Endocrinology*.

Melnick RL. 2019. Commentary on the utility of the National Toxicology Program study on cell phone radiofrequency radiation data for assessing human health risks despite unfounded criticisms aimed at minimizing the findings of adverse health effects. *Environmental Research*.

Miller AB, et al. 2019. Risks to health and well-being from radio-frequency radiation emitted by cell phones and other wireless devices. *Frontiers in Public Health*.

Pall ML. 2018. Wi-Fi is an important threat to human health. *Environmental Research*.

Röösli M, et al. 2019. Brain and salivary gland tumors and mobile phone use: evaluating the evidence from various epidemiological study designs. *Annual Review of Public Health*.

Saliev T, et al. 2019. Biologic effects of non-ionizing electromagnetic fields: two sides of a coin. *Progress in Biophysics and Molecular Biology*.

Santini SJ, et al. 2018. Role of mitochondria in the oxidative stress induced by electromagnetic fields: focus on reproductive systems. *Oxidative Medicine and Cellular Longevity*.

Sato Y, Kojimahara N, Yamaguchi N. 2019. Simulation of the incidence of malignant brain tumors in birth cohorts that started using mobile phones when they first became popular in Japan. *Bioelectromagnetics*.

Schüz J, et al. 2016. Extremely low-frequency magnetic fields and risk of childhood leukemia: a risk assessment by the ARIMMORA consortium. *Bioelectromagnetics*.

Zhang X, Huang WJ, Chen WW. 2016. Microwaves and Alzheimer's disease (review). *Experimental and Therapeutic Medicine*.

Zhi WJ, Wang LF, Hu XJ. 2017. Recent advances in the effects of microwave radiation on brains. *Military Medical Research*.

Electronics

Bellieni CV, et al. 2012. Exposure to electromagnetic fields from laptop use of "laptop" computers. *Archives of Environmental & Occupational Health*.

Mortazavi SAR, et al. 2016. The fundamental reasons why laptop computers should not be used on your lap. *Journal of Biomedical Physics & Engineering*.

van Wel L, et al. 2018. OP VI–2 organ-specific integrative exposure assessment for radio-frequency electromagnetic fields: general population exposure and dose contribution of various sources. *Occupational and Environmental Medicine*.

File Cabinets

Liu Y, Zhu X. 2014. Measurement of formaldehyde and VOCs emissions from wood-based panels with nanomaterial-added melamine-impregnated paper. *Construction and Building Materials*.

Formaldehyde

Ham JE, Siegel PD, Maibach H. 2019. Undeclared formaldehyde levels in patient consumer products: formaldehyde test kit utility. *Cutaneous and Ocular Toxicology*.

Glitter

Karbalaei S, et al. 2018. Occurrence, sources, human health impacts and mitigation of microplastic pollution. *Environmental Science and Pollution Research*.

Markers

Castorina R, et al. 2016. Volatile organic compound emissions from markers used in preschools, schools, and homes. *International Journal of Environmental Analytical Chemistry*.

Duan Y, et al. 2019. Association between phthalate exposure and glycosylated hemoglobin, fasting glucose, and type 2 diabetes mellitus: a case-control study in China. *Science of the Total Environment*.

Fowler BA. 2009. Monitoring of human populations for early markers of cadmium toxicity: a review. *Toxicology and Applied Pharmacology*.

Kandyala R, Raghavendra SPC, Rajasekharan ST. 2010. Xylene: an overview of its health hazards and preventive measures. *Journal of Oral & Maxillofacial Pathology*.

Muchemi SM, Moturi WN, Ogendi GM. 2018. Influence of dry erase ink solvent mixtures on eye irritation. *Journal of Toxicology and Environmental Health Sciences*.

Rajan ST, Malathi N. 2014. Health hazards of xylene: a literature review. *Journal of Clinical and Diagnostic Research*.

Mold

Becher R, et al. 2017. Dampness and moisture problems in Norwegian homes. *International Journal of Environmental Research and Public Health*.

Kontoyiannis DP, Lewis RE. 2015. Treatment principles for the management of mold infections. *Cold Spring Harbor Perspectives in Medicine*.

Park JD, Zheng W. 2012. Human exposure and health effects of inorganic and elemental mercury. *Journal of Preventive Medicine & Public Health*.

Oil Paints

Fowler BA. 2009. Monitoring of human populations for early markers of cadmium toxicity: a review. *Toxicology and Applied Pharmacology*.

Gustin K, et al. 2018. Cadmium exposure and cognitive abilities and behavior at 10 years of age: a prospective cohort study. *Environment International*.

Leyssens L, et al. 2017. Cobalt toxicity in humans—a review of the potential sources and systemic health effects. *Toxicology*.

Ranieri M, et al. 2019. Green olive leaf extract (OLE) provides cytoprotection in renal cells exposed to low doses of cadmium. *PLOS One*.

Satarug S, et al. 2019. The inverse association of glomerular function and urinary β2-MG excretion and its implications for cadmium health risk assessment. *Environmental Research*.

Schoeters G, et al. 2006. Cadmium and children: exposure and health effects. *Acta Paediatrica*.

Wani AL, Ara A, Usmani JA. 2015. Lead toxicity: a review. *Interdisciplinary Toxicology*.

Polyester Resin

Moore MM, Pottenger LH, House-Knight T. 2019. Critical review of styrene genotoxicity focused on the mutagenicity/clastogenicity literature and using current organization of economic cooperation and development guidance. *Environmental and Molecular Mutagenesis*.

Printers

Kowalska J, Szewczyńska M, Pośniak M. 2015. Measurements of chlorinated volatile organic compounds emitted from office printers and photocopiers. *Environmental Science and Pollution Research*.

Pirela SV, et al. 2016. Effects of intratracheally instilled laser printer–emitted engineered nanoparticles in a mouse model: a case study of toxicological implications from nanomaterials released during consumer use. *NanoImpact*.

Solvents

Hedström AK, et al. 2018. Organic solvents and MS susceptibility: interaction with MS risk HLA genes. *Neurology*.

Pajaro-Castro N, Caballero-Gallardo K, Olivero-Verbel J. 2019. Toxicity and expression of oxidative stress genes in *Tribolium castaneum* induced by toluene, xylene, and thinner. *Journal of Toxicology and Environmental Health, Part A*.

Wood Furniture

Qi Y, et al. 2019. Species and release characteristics of VOCs in furniture coating process. *Environmental Pollution*.

CHAPTER NINE: GARAGE AND BASEMENT

Air

Damon SA, et al. 2013. Storm-related carbon monoxide poisoning: an investigation of target audience knowledge and risk behaviors. *Social Marketing Quarterly*.

Howard SG. 2019. Exposure to environmental chemicals and type 1 diabetes: an update. *Journal of Epidemiology & Community Health*.

Mallach G, et al. 2017. Exhaust ventilation in attached garages improves residential indoor air quality. *Indoor Air*.

Mann HS, Crump D, Brown V. 2001. Personal exposure to benzene and the influence of attached and integral garages. *Journal of the Royal Society for the Promotion of Health.*

Rose JJ, et al. 2017. Carbon monoxide poisoning: pathogenesis, management, and future directions of therapy. *American Journal of Respiratory and Critical Care Medicine.*

Antifreeze (Ethylene Glycol)

Wu X, et al. 2017. Antifreeze poisoning: a case report. *Experimental and Therapeutic Medicine.*

Car Air Fresheners

Checkoway H, et al. 2015. Formaldehyde exposure and mortality risks from acute myeloid leukemia and other lymphohematopoietic malignancies in the US National Cancer Institute Cohort study of workers in formaldehyde industries. *Journal of Occupational and Environmental Medicine.*

Zhang L, et al. 2010. Formaldehyde and leukemia: epidemiology, potential mechanisms, and implications for risk assessment. *Environmental and Molecular Mutagenesis.*

Car Exhaust

Bard D, et al. 2014. Traffic-related air pollution and the onset of myocardial infarction: disclosing benzene as a trigger? A small-area case-crossover study. *PLOS One.*

Chen H, et al. 2017. Living near major roads and the incidence of dementia, Parkinson's disease, and multiple sclerosis: a population-based cohort study. *The Lancet.*

Moreno T, et al. 2019. Vehicle interior air quality conditions when travelling by taxi. *Environmental Research.*

Perera F. 2018. Pollution from fossil-fuel combustion is the leading environmental threat to global pediatric health and equity: solutions exist. *International Journal of Environmental Research and Public Health.*

Power MC, et al. 2011. Traffic-related air pollution and cognitive function in a cohort of older men. *Environmental Health Perspectives.*

Suglia SF, et al. 2008. Association between traffic-related black carbon exposure and lung function among urban women. *Environmental Health Perspectives.*

Car Interiors

Brodzik K, et al. 2014. In-vehicle VOCs composition of unconditioned, newly produced cars. *Journal of Environmental Sciences.*

Fang M, et al. 2013. Investigating a novel flame retardant known as V6: measurements in baby products, house dust, and car dust. *Environmental Science & Technology.*

Gibson EA, et al. 2019. Flame retardant exposure assessment: findings from a behavioral intervention study. *Journal of Exposure Science & Environmental Epidemiology.*

Wu Y, et al. 2019. Children's car seats contain legacy and novel flame retardants. *Environmental Science & Technology Letters.*

Furnaces

Dietz E, et al. 2016. [Carbon monoxide poisoning by a heating system.] Article in German. *Archiv Für Kriminologie.*

Glue

Roth S, Fell AKM. 2016. Multiple subcutaneous granulomas and severe rhinitis after intradermal deposition of epoxy: a case report. *Journal of Occupational Medicine and Toxicology.*

Insecticides

Eddleston M, Chowdhury FR. 2016. Pharmacological treatment of organo-phosphorus insecticide poisoning: the old and the (possible) new. *British Journal of Clinical Pharmacology.*

Paint

Delgado-Saborit JM, et al. 2009. Model development and validation of personal exposure to volatile organic compound concentrations. *Environmental Health Perspectives.*

Kwon JW, et al. 2018. Exposure to volatile organic compounds and airway inflammation. *Environmental Health.*

Scélo G, et al. 2009. Household exposure to paint and petroleum solvents, chromosomal translocations, and the risk of childhood leukemia. *Environmental Health Perspectives.*

Paint Thinners

Singh R, Vinayagam S, Vajifdar H. 2012. Methemoglobinemia as a result of accidental lacquer thinner poisoning. *Indian Journal of Critical Care Medicine.*

Pesticides

Ganapathy S, et al. 2019. Chronic low dose arsenic exposure preferentially perturbs mitotic phase of the cell cycle. *Genes & Cancer.*

Li Y, et al. 2016. Chronic arsenic poisoning probably caused by arsenic-based pesticides: findings from an investigation study of a household. *International Journal of Environmental Research and Public Health.*

Nicolopoulou-Stamati P, et al. 2016. Chemical pesticides and human health: the urgent need for a new concept in agriculture. *Frontiers in Public Health.*

Roy JS, et al. 2018. Substantial evidences indicate that inorganic arsenic is a genotoxic carcinogen: a review. *Toxicological Research.*

Radon

Garcia-Rodriguez JA. 2018. Radon gas—the hidden killer: what is the role of family doctors? *Canadian Family Physician.*

Rust Remover

Bajraktarova-Valjakova E, et. al. 2018. Hydrofluoric acid: burns and systemic toxicity, protective measures, immediate and hospital medical treatment. *Open Access Macedonian Journal of Medical Sciences.*

Solvents

Lash LH. 2019. Environmental and genetic factors influencing kidney toxicity. *Seminars in Nephrology.*

Lee KM, et al. 2019. Alterations in immune and renal biomarkers among workers occupationally exposed to low levels of trichloroethylene below current regulatory standards. *Occupational & Environmental Medicine.*

Pajaro-Castro N, Caballero-Gallardo K, Olivero-Verbel J. 2019. Toxicity and expression of oxidative stress genes in *Tribolium castaneum* induced by toluene, xylene, and thinner. *Journal of Toxicology and Environmental Health, Part A.*

Pastor Jimeno JC, Coco Martin RM. 2017. The acute toxicity problem with some perfluorooctanes. *Archivos de la Sociedad Española de Oftalmología.*

Spray Paint

West GH, et al. 2019. Exposure to airborne nano-titanium dioxide during airless spray painting and sanding. *Journal of Occupational and Environmental Hygiene.*

Tires

Kole PJ, et al. 2017. Wear and tear of tyres: a stealthy source of microplastics in the environment. *International Journal of Environmental Research and Public Health.*

Turpentine

Güzel A, Açıkgöz M. 2015. A lethal danger in the home: turpentine poisoning. *The Turkish Journal of Pediatrics.*

Rahimi HR, et al. 2015. Clinical and biochemical analysis of acute paint thinner intoxication in adults: a retrospective descriptive study. *Toxicology Mechanisms and Methods.*

Windshield Wiper Fluid

Moon CS. 2017. Estimations of the lethal and exposure doses for representative methanol symptoms in humans. *Annals of Occupational and Environmental Medicine.*

CHAPTER TEN: YARD AND GARDEN

Barbecue Grill Fumes

Lao JY, et al. 2018. Importance of dermal absorption of polycyclic aromatic hydrocarbons derived from barbecue fumes. *Environmental Science & Technology.*

Bug Repellents

Asadollahi A, et al. 2019. Effectiveness of plant-based repellents against different *Anopheles* species: a systematic review. *Malaria Journal.*

Lee, MY. 2018. Essential oils as repellents against arthropods. *BioMed Research International.*

Sanghong R, et al. 2015. Remarkable repellency of *Ligusticum sinense* (Umbelliferae), a herbal alternative against laboratory populations of *Anopheles minimus* and *Aedes aegypti* (Diptera: Culicidae). *Malaria Journal.*

Zhu JJ, et al. 2018. Better than DEET repellent compounds derived from coconut oil. *Scientific Reports.*

Fire Pits

Sansom GT, et al. 2018. Domestic exposures to polycyclic aromatic hydrocarbons in a Houston, Texas, environmental justice neighborhood. *Environmental Justice.*

Abdel-Shafy HI, Mansour MSM. 2016. A review on polycyclic aromatic hydrocarbons: source, environmental impact, effect on human health and remediation. *Egyptian Journal of Petroleum.*

Idowu O, et al. 2019. Beyond the obvious: environmental health implications of polar polycyclic aromatic hydrocarbons. *Environment International.*

Garden Hoses

Ecology Center. 2016. Garden Hose Study.

Sathyanarayana S, et al. 2013. Unexpected results in a randomized dietary trial to reduce phthalate and bisphenol A exposures. *Journal of Exposure Science & Environmental Epidemiology.*

Herbicides

Davoren MJ, Schiestl RH. 2018. Glyphosate-based herbicides and cancer risk: a post-IARC decision review of potential mechanisms, policy and avenues of research. *Carcinogenesis.*

Defarge N, de Vendômois JS, Séralini GE. 2018. Toxicity of formulants and heavy metals in glyphosate-based herbicides and other pesticides. *Toxicology Reports.*

Gillezeau C, et al. 2019. The evidence of human exposure to glyphosate: a review. *Environmental Health.*

Hayes HM, et al. 1991. Case-control study of canine malignant lymphoma: positive association with dog owner's use of 2,4-dichlorophenoxyacetic acid herbicides. *JNCI: Journal of the National Cancer Institute.*

International Agency for Research on Cancer (IARC). 2015. IARC monographs evaluate DDT, lindane, and 2,4-D. Press release.

Kubsad D, et al. 2019. Assessment of glyphosate induced epigenetic transgenerational inheritance of pathologies and sperm epimutations: generational toxicology. *Scientific Reports*.

Mills PJ, et al. 2017. Excretion of the herbicide glyphosate in older adults between 1993 and 2016. *JAMA*.

Pham TH, et al. 2019. Perinatal exposure to glyphosate and a glyphosate-based herbicide affect spermatogenesis in mice. *Toxicological Sciences*.

Takashima-Uebelhoer BB, et al. 2012. Household chemical exposures and the risk of canine malignant lymphoma, a model for human non-Hodgkin's lymphoma. *Environmental Research*.

Zhang L, et al. 2019. Exposure to glyphosate-based herbicides and risk for non-Hodgkin lymphoma: a meta-analysis and supporting evidence. *Mutation Research/Reviews in Mutation Research*.

Plastic Pools/Swim Toys

Dodson RE, et al. 2012. Endocrine disruptors and asthma-associated chemicals in consumer products. *Environmental Health Perspectives*.

Wiedmer C, Buettner A. 2018. Quantification of organic solvents in aquatic toys and swimming learning devices and evaluation of their influence on the smell properties of the corresponding products. *Analytical and Bioanalytical Chemistry*.

Play Sets

King CMD, et al. 2019. Long-term leaching of arsenic from pressure-treated playground structures in the northeastern United States. *Science of the Total Environment*.

Porch and Deck Wood

Costa M. 2019. Review of arsenic toxicity, speciation and polyadenylation of canonical histones. *Toxicology and Applied Pharmacology*.

Gress J, et al. 2015. Cleaning-induced arsenic mobilization and chromium oxidation from CCA-wood deck: potential risk to children. *Environment International*.

Gress J. 2015. Residential exposures to arsenic and hexavalent chromium from CCA-wood. PhD dissertation, University of Florida.

Soil

Li Z. 2018. Health risk characterization of maximum legal exposures for persistent organic pollutant (POP) pesticides in residential soil: an analysis. *Journal of Environmental Management*.

Myers JP, et al. 2016. Concerns over use of glyphosate-based herbicides and risks associated with exposures: a consensus statement. *Environmental Health*.

Nezat CA, Hatch SA, Uecker T. 2017. Heavy metal content in urban residential and park soils: a case study in Spokane, Washington, USA. *Applied Geochemistry*.

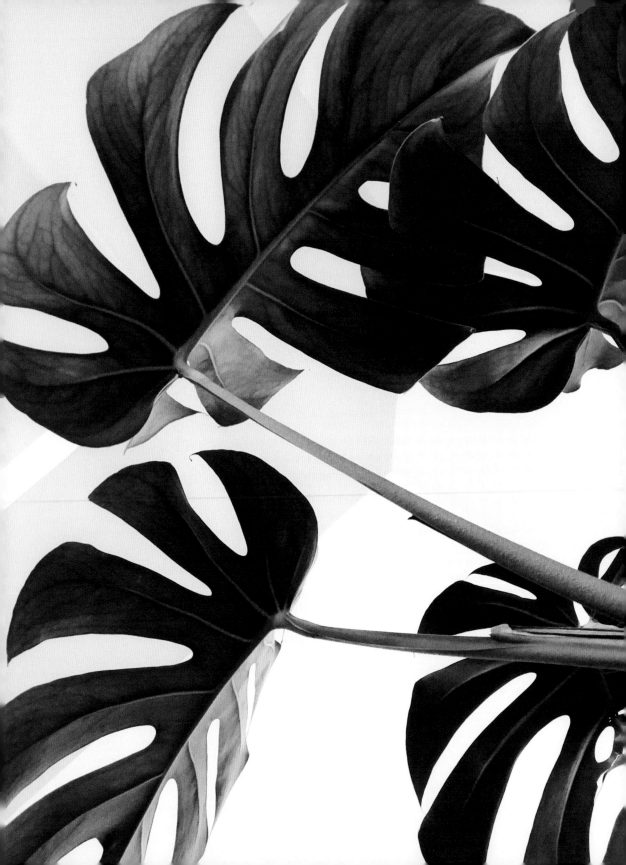

ACKNOWLEDGMENTS

I am forever grateful to Riley Revallier for her dedication to this book; she reviewed thousands of studies, tested numerous products and formulas, and spent countless hours searching out the most effective eco-centered resources for our readers.

A special thank you to Helen Thompson of HelenMilan.com, who supplied her own personal photographs of many of my favorite eco-lifestyle objects and tools. I am such a huge fan of Helen Milan that I have almost all of the items from their online store in my home now. Their curated collection of natural and nontoxic cleaning brushes and brooms features well-made products from across the globe. These quality items appear in photos and paintings throughout the book.

I am so grateful to my mother, Linda Landkammer, who has been living simply and in tune with the environment for decades and is my compass. Thanks also to Liz Bevilacqua, my thoughtful editor; Alethea Morrison and Michaela Jebb, for their artistic direction; my literary agent, Linda Konner; Brad Matsen, my Port Townsend editor; and Todd Masters, who spent many hours cleaning up my messy paintings in Photoshop; Tom and Merrilee Gomez for inspiring a natural lifestyle all those years ago; Jim Banholzer for sharing his medical case for use in this book; and Sebastian "Seb" Eggert for lending his expertise on electromagnetic fields. With great appreciation to Tara Hubbard and Eric Kestner for the emotional support during the many long months of research; Tony Chace for all of those meetings to discuss the scope of the book; Rob Dunn for his comments on the microbes in house dust; and Robin Dodson for her expertise on the chemical nature of house dust.

INDEX

Page numbers in **bold** font indicate charts and tables. Page numbers in *italics* indicate images.

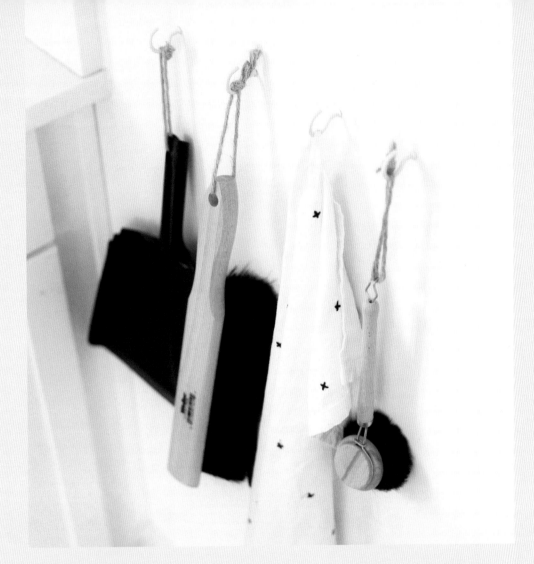

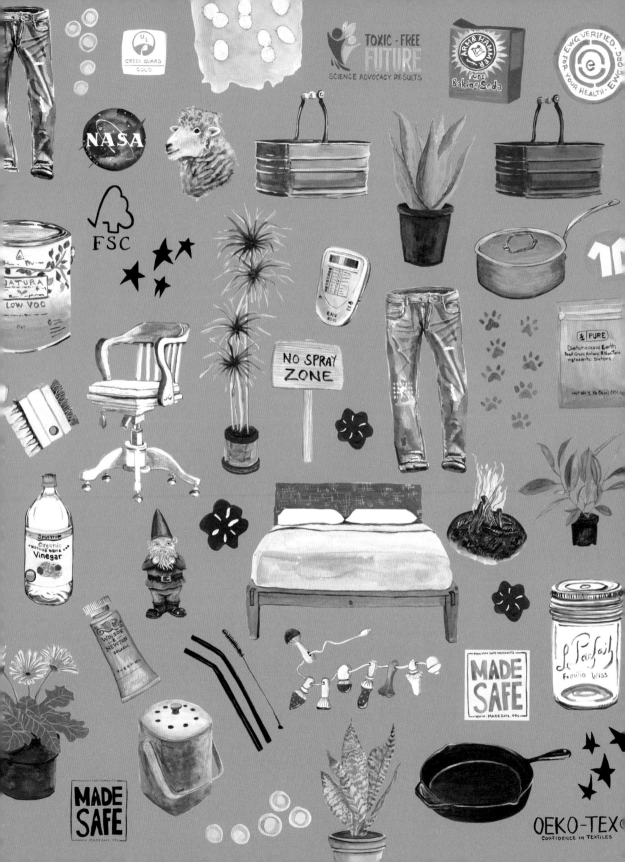